I LOST 140 POUNDS IN A YEAR

TIM WEISS

ISBN 978-1-956001-27-3 (paperback)
ISBN 978-1-956001-28-0 (digital)

Printed in the United States of America

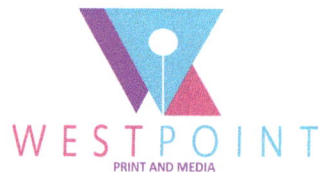

WESTPOINT
PRINT AND MEDIA

Preface

I've been very overweight for many years. There was nothing medically wrong with me and no doctor told me that I had to lose weight. I just woke up one morning and decided I needed to lose weight and change my eating habits. I set myself a target... to lose all my excess weight in one year. I wasn't sure if I could do that, but I needed a target to go for.

If I failed to lose all my excess weight, I would certainly be well on my way to achieving this by the end of the year.

I was like most people, I ate out a lot, got takeaways (takeouts), had readymade meals and prepackaged foods. This type of food is laced with calories, chemicals and preservatives that you don't need or want. So I decided to change. I started preparing my own meals. I also learnt how to make homemade sauces from natural ingredients. These homemade sauces added so much taste to my meals, and everything in these sauces were from natural ingredients.

When you read this book you're not reading about a complicated diet; it's a lifestyle change. The way you have been eating has made you overweight, so you need to look at the food you're eating and change your habits. Get into a healthier way of thinking. You will benefit greatly from this.

On December 12th I made up my mind to change, to lose all my excess weight. I knew at first this would be hard, but I was determined. I weighed myself and I was 24 Stone 5 pounds that's 341 pounds.

Some of you will say you can't cook. Some meals are as easy as putting on your shoes.

Some will say they don't have time to cook their own meals. Well those people need to ask themselves another question, just how much do they really want to lose weight?

If you want this weight loss journey to be successful, you're going to have to really want to change and really want to lose weight. Be prepared to make lifestyle changes that will benefit you forever.

I hope you enjoy reading this book.

Chapter One

Starting Out

So you want to lose weight? Don't we all. This book is not a diet book. It's not complicated in any way. There is no magic formula. It is a simple way we eat our food and how we can all lose weight by changing our eating habits.

Get into a routine of making and preparing your own meals using natural ingredients. That's all you need to do to lose weight.

I would like to point out that in my recipes I'll have the English version and American version next to each other. For example, salad cream (miracle whip).

The Foods You Can Eat

- Any meat and poultry; just cut off any excess fat from the meat. You can do this before or after cooking. If you choose to have minced meat (ground beef), make sure it's 5% fat.
- Any fish.
- Fresh, frozen or canned vegetables.
- Fruit that is fresh or frozen.
- Beans, peas and pulses.
- Tinned tuna or salmon.
- Potatoes are great to have in your meals and are perfectly okay. Homemade chips (French fries) are great.
- Tinned baked beans and tinned tomatoes are great and very good.
- Plain couscous, rice, and pasta are great to have with your meat and vegetables.
- Eggs are fantastic, full of protein and very versatile.

- Soy sauce, Worcester sauce, oyster sauce, marmite, mustard, fat free dressings, Canderel (Splenda), tomato puree.
- Any herbs and spices.
- Any stock like beef, vegetable or chicken.
- Vinegar, salt and pepper.
- Drinks: water (plain, tap, mineral or spring), tea, coffee, low calorie fizzy drinks. No added sugar cordials, Bovril (beef drink).
- Try to avoid bread completely if you can. But if you do use bread use wholemeal (wholegrain).
- Tomato ketchup, mayonnaise and salad cream (miracle whip) are okay in small doses.
- Milk: try and use skimmed milk if you can. Orange milk is okay to use, but not in great quantities.
- Fat free yogurts (unflavored yogurt)
- Quark (a tasteless yogurt style cheese) is fantastic to use in cooking.
- Cheese is okay. Try and use 25g of cheese per day. Or 50g of reduced fat cheese.
- If you do use butter or margarine just look for reduced fat.
- Use a low calorie cooking spray (Pam Original Cooking Spray fat free). You can still fry all your food, just use low calorie cooking spray

A lot of the foods you see in the shops are totally loaded with chemicals and preservatives that we don't want or need, and of course packed with calories. So please be vigilant.

You can add lots of flavor to all your meals by just adding a few herbs or spices in the ingredients.

Or, you can make a homemade sauce.

Homemade sauce can be made from curry powder, chili powder, or mustard powder. With these powders you just add water. Also you can add garlic and or ginger. You can also add mushrooms, onions and peppers. This makes a tremendous sauce for your meals.

Or you can use passata (tomato sauce) or tinned tomatoes mixed with herbs and spices and add soy sauce, Worcester sauce, tomato puree or balsamic vinegar.

Another idea is to get an egg, whisk it up, and cover a couple of chicken legs. Get chicken seasoning mixed with plain flour (all purpose flour) and pour it over the chicken legs. Then put these in the oven at Gas Mark 6 - 400f for thirty-five minutes. These are a few ideas for making a homemade sauce.

I LOST 140 POUNDS IN A YEAR

You can make your homemade sauce as mild or as hot or even as spicy as you like. It's all down to personal taste.

However, because you making your own sauce up from natural ingredients, you know exactly what's in your meal. By doing this you're making a very healthy well balanced meal that tastes great. What more could you want from your meal?

You can Google homemade sauces to give you some new ideas. Just check the ingredients they use. Obviously once you become more experienced from making your own sauces you can pick and choose which ingredients you prefer. There are dozens and dozens of homemade sauces you can make. Adding homemade sauces is excellent. It adds lots of great taste to all your meals.

So you can make yourself a big meal, with lots of flavor and virtually no calories. What more do you want in your meals?

It's Not How Much You Eat, But It's What You Eat That Matters

During the day I would drink two or three litres of water. At night when I got home, I'd drink mainly black coffee or herbal tea and the odd can of a diet fizzy drink.

I love fruit and I had lots and lots of fruit to eat every day. I didn't find this a chore because I actually like fruit. So I ate lots and lots of fruit every day. I never went hungry during the day so this made it easier to carry on losing weight.

I would like to point out from the outset I'm not a dietician, a nutritionist, or a medical professional. I'm a normal guy who lost a lot of weight within one year.

I'd also like to specify that going to the gym is not essential. Going to the gym does not help you lose weight. It gets you more fit, stronger and healthier.

I think it's very important to plan your meals a week in advance. This gets you into a routine and it's healthy to get into a routine. Planning your meals ahead is good because you know exactly what you're going to eat on any particular day.

The Foods You Must Avoid

- All bread… if you must have bread use wholemeal (wholegrain) bread; it's okay to have 2 slices of wholemeal (wholegrain) a day or a wholemeal (wholegrain) roll.
- Personally I completely cut bread and butter out of my life altogether.

- Butter and margarine.
- Any prepackaged food, any processed food, any readymade meals. All these foods are packed with chemicals and preservatives you don't want or need and have loads of unwanted calories in them.
- Any takeaway (takeout).

Take notice and read all readymade meals and prepackaged meals. There are certain meals out there specifically made for people trying to lose weight. So not all readymade meals are bad for you.

Obviously avoid chocolate, crisps (potato chips), cakes, biscuits (cookies), sweets and everything like that.

Yes it's okay to have a treat now and again, but having a treat will slow your weight loss down. If you do have a treat it's okay; just be careful and monitor all treats.

The Old Adage, You Are What You Eat Is So True

I go shopping every week; I look at what everyone buys: tons of premade food and meals and lots of prepackaged readymade foods. Do you actually know how many calories are in this food and all the chemicals and preservatives they put in it? Do you wonder why you put weight on?

It's best if you plan your meals a week ahead. I do my weekly shopping on a Saturday, so I plan all my meals on a Thursday or Friday. So when I go shopping I buy all the natural ingredients I need.

Get into the habit of planning your meal and cooking all your meals. Yes I know at first it's hard, but please stick with it. You will benefit so much by doing this and you can lose weight.

Please don't use the excuse that you don't get time to cook your meals. If you do say this, ask yourself another question, how much do you really want to lose weight? Make time to cook your meals. You will benefit from it.

It's very hard to lose weight, but to successfully lose weight is something that you really want to do. This book is trying to show you how easy it is to lose weight. Cooking your own meals is also cheaper than buying prepackaged foods.

This book is all about a change in lifestyle.

This is not a diet book. I'm showing you how to change your lifestyle in how you eat your food.

You Are What You Eat

After a short time you can lose weight and you will be buying smaller clothes. This will make you feel so much better. People will start to come up to you and say, "Have you lost weight? You're looking good." All this can happen fairly quickly. You will see the benefit of cooking your own meals in a short time.

I know from personal experience that there is no better feeling inside than when people came up to me and complimented me on how good I was looking because I was losing weight. This spurred me on to keep up cooking my own meals.

I've put in a few recipes in this book. Every meal in this book you can change by adding herbs and spices or adding a homemade sauce. The choices of homemade sauces are endless, and you can experiment in making new sauces. It's vital that you use natural ingredients for your sauces. By doing this, you know exactly what's in the meal you're cooking. I'm trying to show you that you can really do things with your meals to make them much more exciting to eat.

I have a very sweet tooth which is not a good thing to have. I have put in two recipes that helped me with my sweet tooth. I would have one of these sweet tasting meals every week. I would satisfy my sweet tooth and not put any weight on.

For some of us, it's a time thing. We don't have time to do this or cook that. So we bung something in the oven or microwave and eat. You must ask yourself another question, just how much do you want to lose weight? If you really want to lose weight you will make the time to cook yourself a good meal.

I've lost 10 Stone (140 pounds) in one year. I've changed my lifestyle by preparing my own foods. I've seen how much weight I've lost and how much better I feel inside. I will never go back to the way I used to eat my food. I'm certain if you all changed the way you prepare and eat your food you will all change, and all of you will make time to prepare and cook your food. You will make the time up from somewhere.

This book is about a lifestyle change. It's going to try and show you how to make your own meals, with natural ingredients. You can change the taste of your food by adding herbs or spices or adding a homemade sauce.

"I can't cook," some of you will say. Okay. Get a fillet of fish, put salt and herbs on it, wrap it in tin foil and put it in the oven Gas Mark 7 - 425f for thirty minutes. Prepare some salad. Job done it's that easy. Or get a lamb chop, pour seasoning on it, put it in the oven for twenty-five minutes, and make sure you turn the chop over after twelve minutes. Cut up some fresh vegetables and boil, Depending on what vegetables you are using, boil them for five minutes to fifteen minutes. Again, an easy cooking job. That's just two easy to cook meals; there are hundreds just as easy. So "I can't cook" is not a valid excuse.

By preparing your own meals with natural ingredients you are eating very healthily. You can lose weight and add years to your life. Surely this alone is a good enough reason to want to change.

Packaged and prepared meals cost you considerably more than cooking with raw ingredients at home. Preparing meals at home can save you money.

Preparing meals at home allows you to control the amount of salt and oils you use in your recipes. This in turn reduces the possibility of weight gain and clogged arteries.

Taking the time to plan your weekly menu not only helps to save time and money, but also provides a way to create meals with a balance of protein, carbohydrates and fat, plus all the essential vitamins and minerals needed for the adult's and child's body. When eating balanced meals, your body feels much better. You can lose weight and that will make you fill so much better.

Plan Your Meals a Week Ahead

It will take you a little time to think about eating differently, but after a very short time of preparing your own meals you can lose some weight. Get into smaller clothes and you will fill so much better about it. You haven't actually done anything except eat differently. You haven't gone to the gym four times a week or joined and paid some slimming club money and you haven't had an operation.

So please think about it. Plan your week's food ahead. Go shopping and buy all the food you need with natural ingredients. Getting yourself into a routine of planning ahead is very good for your mind.

When you prepare your own meals you can choose how much fat or carbohydrates you have in your food.

Yes, treat yourself now and again, nothing wrong with that. But please just monitor your treats carefully.

Okay just a little recap.

- You don't need to join a slimming club.
- You don't need to go to the gym four times a week.
- You don't need an operation.
- All you need to do is to plan your meals in advance and cook them from scratch.
- You will save money by buying fresh food.
- You can lose weight and feel better for it. That's a promise.

If you're going to use the lifestyle change in your eating habits as a diet that's okay. That's exactly what I did. I used this new way of eating to lose weight, but you have to be strong and remain on track. You can soon lose weight and see the difference in a short period of time. All I ask you to do is when you have lost all your weight, continue to eat this way, but have the odd treat here and there. This will maintain your new weight and you will not put weight back on.

Before you start keep one pair of jeans, or skirt and a polo shirt. Just keep these in a drawer somewhere. After a couple of months try them on again and see how much weight you have lost. This method is a great inspiration to keep up the good work that you're doing.

It's not how much you eat; it's what you eat that matters.

Chapter Two

Stage One

I need to point out immediately. I changed the way I eat my food December 12, 2014. I started to plan and prepare all my meals. It was a lifestyle change for me, but I called it a diet. Calling it a diet helped me to concentrate and keep on track. I had set myself a goal to lose all my excess fat in one year. I wasn't sure if I could do that, but that was my target.

From day one I cut out bread and butter completely. Yes, I used to love my sandwiches, but sandwiches got me fat. So I cut out bread completely. I just told myself, it's only for a short time Tim.

After one month I had lost 2 Stone (28 pounds). I felt so much better. The month had flown past and I was already in smaller clothes. I can't tell you in only a few words how good this made me feel. All I had done was prepare my own meals.

I knew that on this weight loss journey I would need to change my eating patterns. I knew this had to be done, to stop me becoming bored or my body getting used to the food. So I knew I needed to make several changes on my weight loss journey. So let's call this stage one.

All my life I've never had a breakfast except on Sunday mornings. So I thought, okay, let's start having a breakfast each morning. After all, it's a lifestyle change. So I looked up a few healthy breakfasts to eat. I thought I'd have a different breakfast each morning.

There is a wonderful thing you can use that is very low in calories. If you like frying your food, use a low calorie cooking spray for cooking curries where olive oil is needed. It's absolutely fantastic. You can use as much low calorie cooking spray as you like. It has virtually no calories in it.

So for example, one of my breakfasts is three rashers of fried bacon, two fried eggs and a tin of beans. This is extremely healthy, filling and very tasty. What more can you want for any meal? Low calorie cooking spray is a must in your kitchen cupboard.

You Are What You Eat.

Let me give you a few breakfasts I had to start off with. All of them are filling, tasty and healthy with virtually no calories in them.

Jamaican Jerk Chicken

Ingredients

1 large chicken fillet

onions, peppers, mushrooms

3 tbsp. jamaican jerk seasoning

6 tbsp. canderal (splenda)

1/2 cup water

1/2 cup rice

low calorie cooking spray

Method

Cut the chicken into bite size pieces and pan fry them in low calorie cooking spray.

Add 3 tbsp of jamaican jerk seasoning and 6 tbsp of canderal (splenda) with ½ a cup of water and cook in a wok with the chicken.

Cut the onions, peppers and mushrooms into pieces and pan fry them in plenty of low calorie cooking spray. Add the vegetables to the chicken and keep cooking for about 20 mins.

Put the 1/2 cup of rice into a saucepan of water and boil for 20 minutes.

This is a very tasty meal.

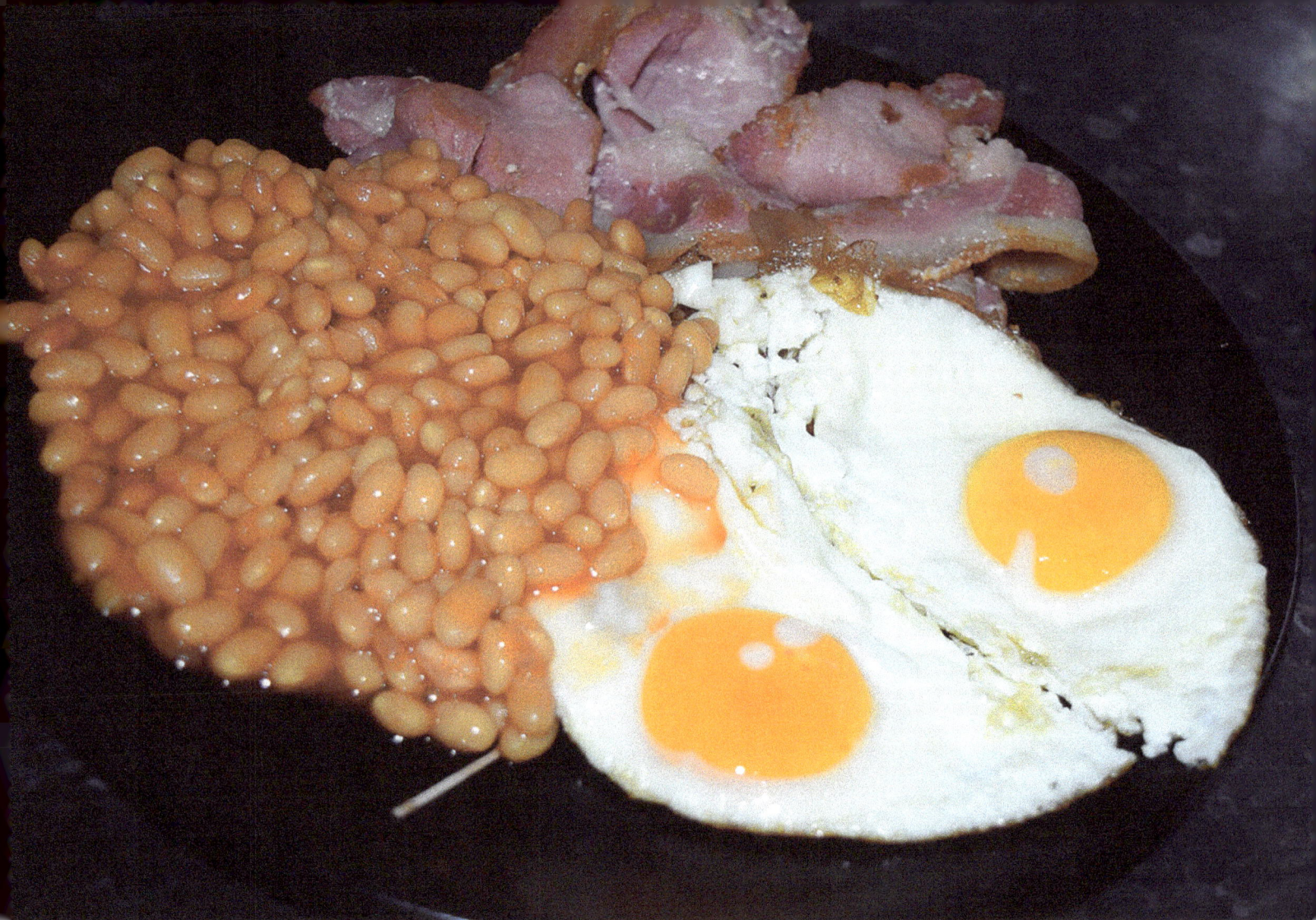

My Breakfast

Ingredients

- 4 rashers of bacon
- 2 eggs
- low calorie cooking spray
- tin of baked beans
- you can add mushrooms or tomatoes to this if you wanted.

Method

1. fry the rashers of bacon in low calorie cooking spray.
2. fry the eggs in low calorie cooking spray.
3. microwave the baked beans for two and a half minutes

A very filling, tasty breakfast that is perfect for weight loss.

I had this breakfast every weekend for a whole year. It's very healthy; the bacon, eggs and beans are packed with protein. I fried the bacon and eggs with low calorie cooking spray.

Bacon, eggs and beans are full of protein and that is healthy. You're frying the bacon and eggs with low calorie cooking spray which is excellent. There are virtually no calories in this meal.

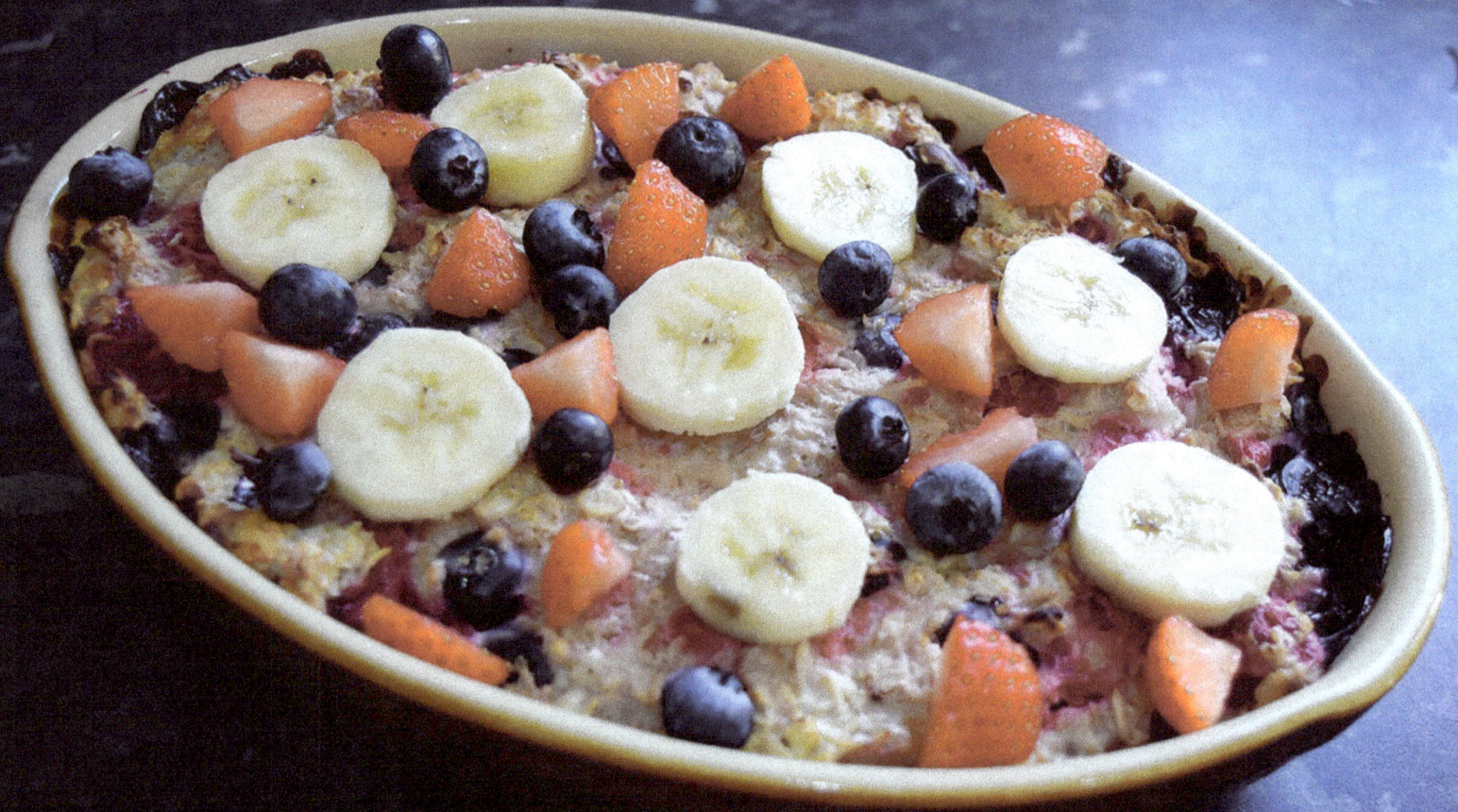

Baked Oats

Ingredients

- 35g plain porridge oats (cooked oatmeal)
- 5 tbsp. canderel (splenda)
- 1 small egg
- 90g of fat free natural yogurt (unflavored yogurt)
- a few drops of vanilla extract
- 30g raspberries
- 30g strawberries
- 30g blueberries

Method

1. Preheat your oven to Gas Mark 6 – 400f.

2. Mix the porridge (cooked oatmeal), sweetener, egg, yogurt (unflavored yogurt), vanilla extract and raspberries in a bowl and stir well.

3. Transfer the mixture to a small oven-proof dish and bake in the oven for thirty-five minutes, or until browned.

4. Serve with whatever fruit you like. I have to be honest with you, I have this very often; I use raspberries, strawberries, blueberries and bananas. I use low fat natural yogurt (unflavored yogurt) with it in the mixture. Then I use fat free natural yogurt (unflavored yogurt) with it as I eat it. It tastes absolutely gorgeous. It's very healthy and tastes great; what more could you want?

You can have this as a breakfast, an afternoon snack or as a desert after a meal.

In this mixture, I put in 100g of porridge oats (cooked oatmeal). This lasted for a few days. I just multiply everything by three.

I will be honest with you. I had this a lot—almost weekly. I have a sweet tooth and you can add more sweeteners to add sweetness to this. Canderel (Splenda) has virtually zero calories, so it doesn't matter how much you use. If you're like me and have a sweet tooth, then cook this.

I used fat free natural yogurt (unflavored yogurt) (see photo) and had that with baked oats. I cannot tell you only in a few words how good this tastes… and it's healthy.

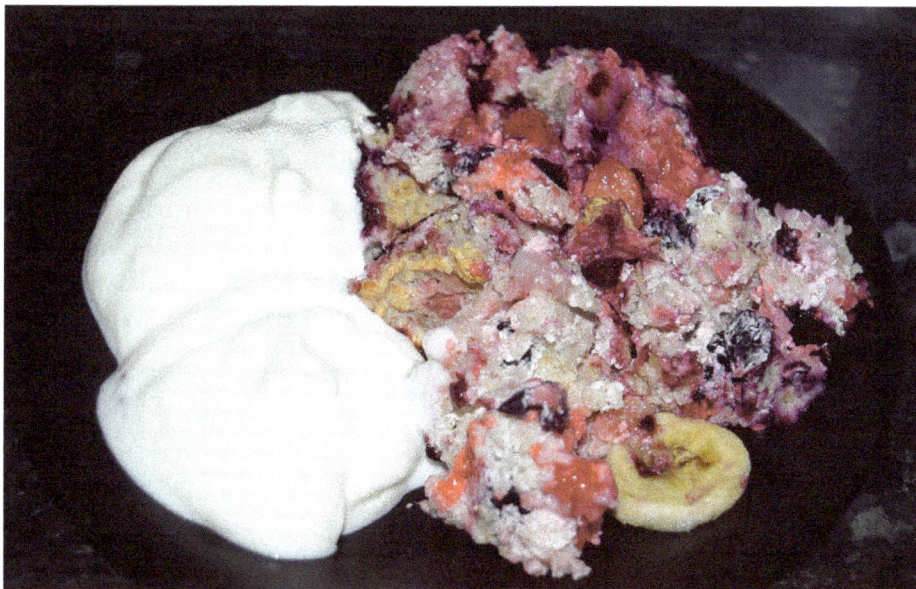

Eggs with Peppers, Spinach and Tomato

Ingredients

- 400g new potatoes, thickly sliced
- low calorie cooking spray
- 1 onion, finely chopped
- 1 garlic clove, finely chopped
- 1 orange pepper, deseeded and cut into small pieces
- 400g can cannellini beans, drained and rinsed
- 400g can chopped tomatoes with herbs
- 300ml passata (tomato sauce)
- 12 tbsp. worcester sauce (bold steak sauce)
- Salt and freshly ground black pepper
- 100g spinach
- 4 large eggs
- A handful of basil, to garnish

Method

1. Boil the potatoes for a few minutes, or until just tender. Drain well.
2. Meanwhile, spray a large frying pan with low calorie cooking spray and place over a medium-high heat. Add the onion, garlic and pepper and stir-fry for a few minutes until softened.
3. Stir in the potatoes and beans, and then add the tomatoes, passata (tomato sauce) and Worcester sauce to taste. Season and simmer for ten to twelve minutes, or until thickened.
4. Stir through the spinach and allow it to wilt. Make four shallow indents in the mixture and crack an egg into each one. Cover and cook gently for five minutes, or place under a medium-hot grill, until the eggs are set to your liking. Add a twist of black pepper and serve garnished with basil leaves.

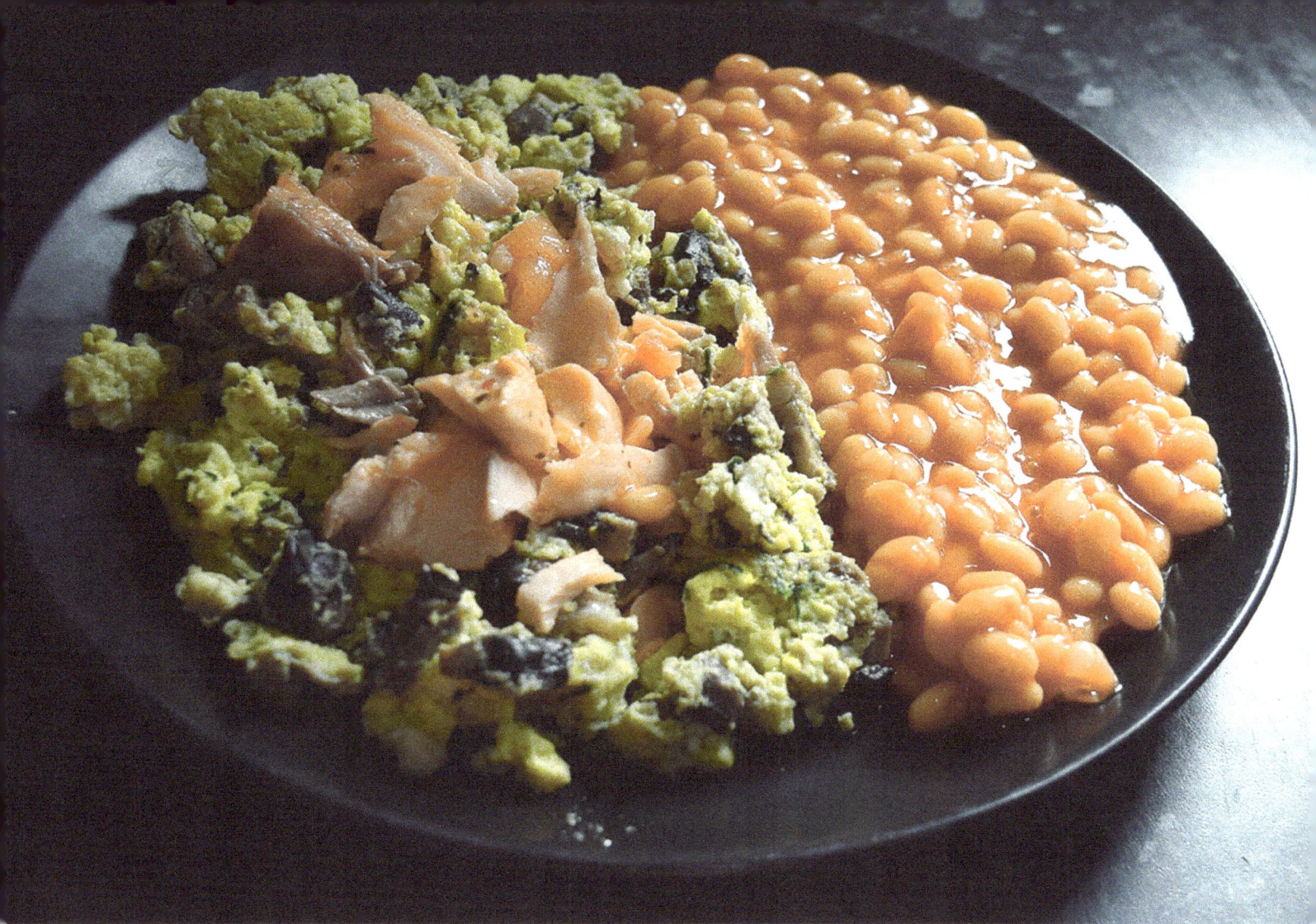

Salmon and Scrambled Eggs

Ingredients

- 4 large eggs
- a few sprigs of fresh dill or chives, finely chopped
- salt and freshly ground black pepper
- wholemeal (wholegrain) roll
- 250g pack smoked salmon
- ½ cup of double cream (heavy cream)

Method

1. Lightly whisk the eggs with the dill or chives and some seasoning.
2. Preheat a non-stick frying pan. Add the herby egg mixture and continue to cook slowly until the eggs are scrambled to your liking. You can either mix in the salmon or just place the salmon on top.
3. Cut the wholemeal (wholegrain) roll in half and put the egg and salmon on top.

I added some mushrooms to this, but it's basically scrambled eggs, so you add ham, bacon, onions as well. It's all down to personal preference.

This is a great afternoon snack, as you can see from the photos you can have it on a wholemeal roll (wholegrain roll) or have it with beans. It's very healthy packed with protein and very healthy.

I did tell people not to have bread at all, but if you do have bread make sure it's wholemeal (wholegrain bread), as I did in this meal. I had a wholemeal (wholegrain) roll perfectly okay.

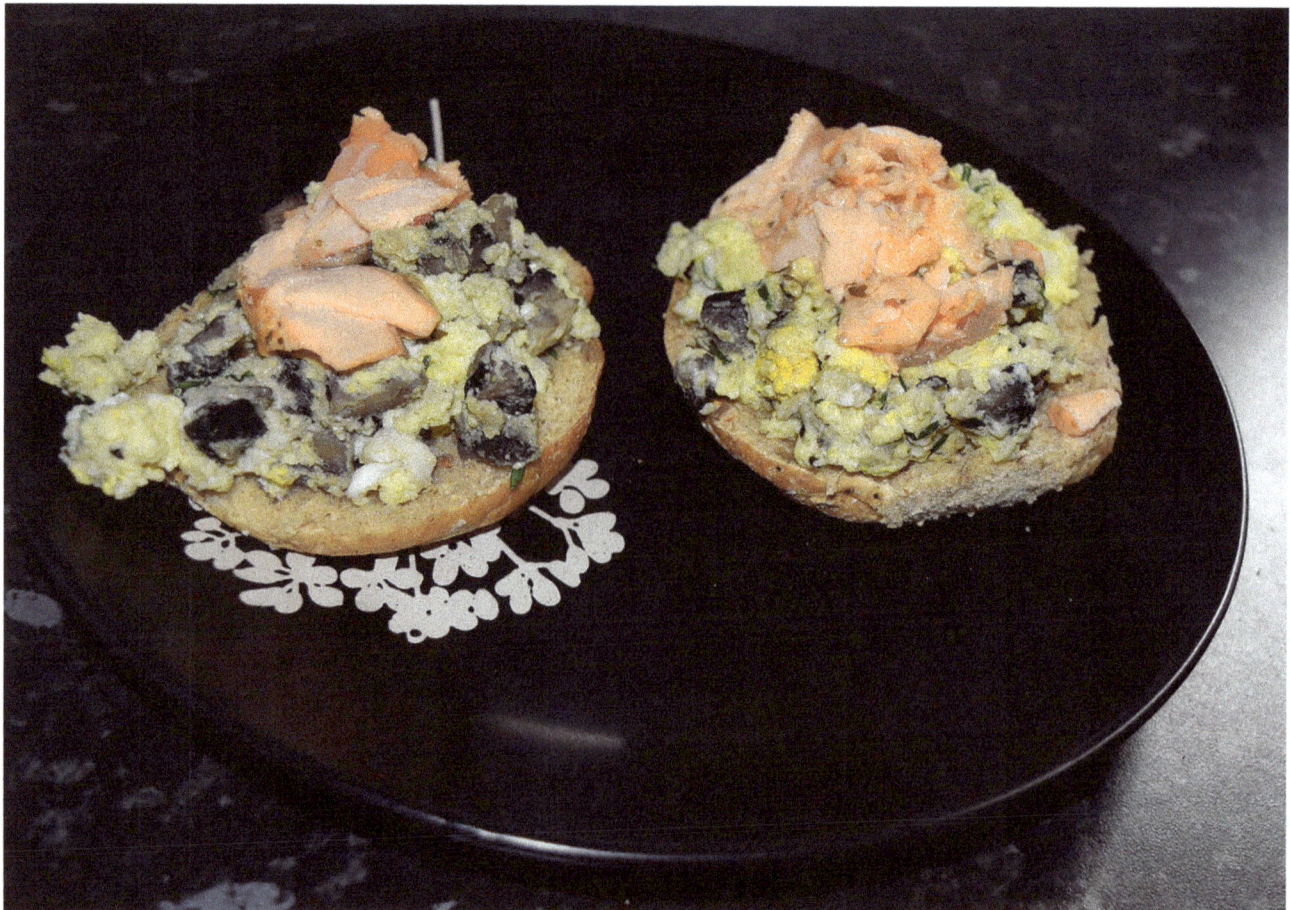

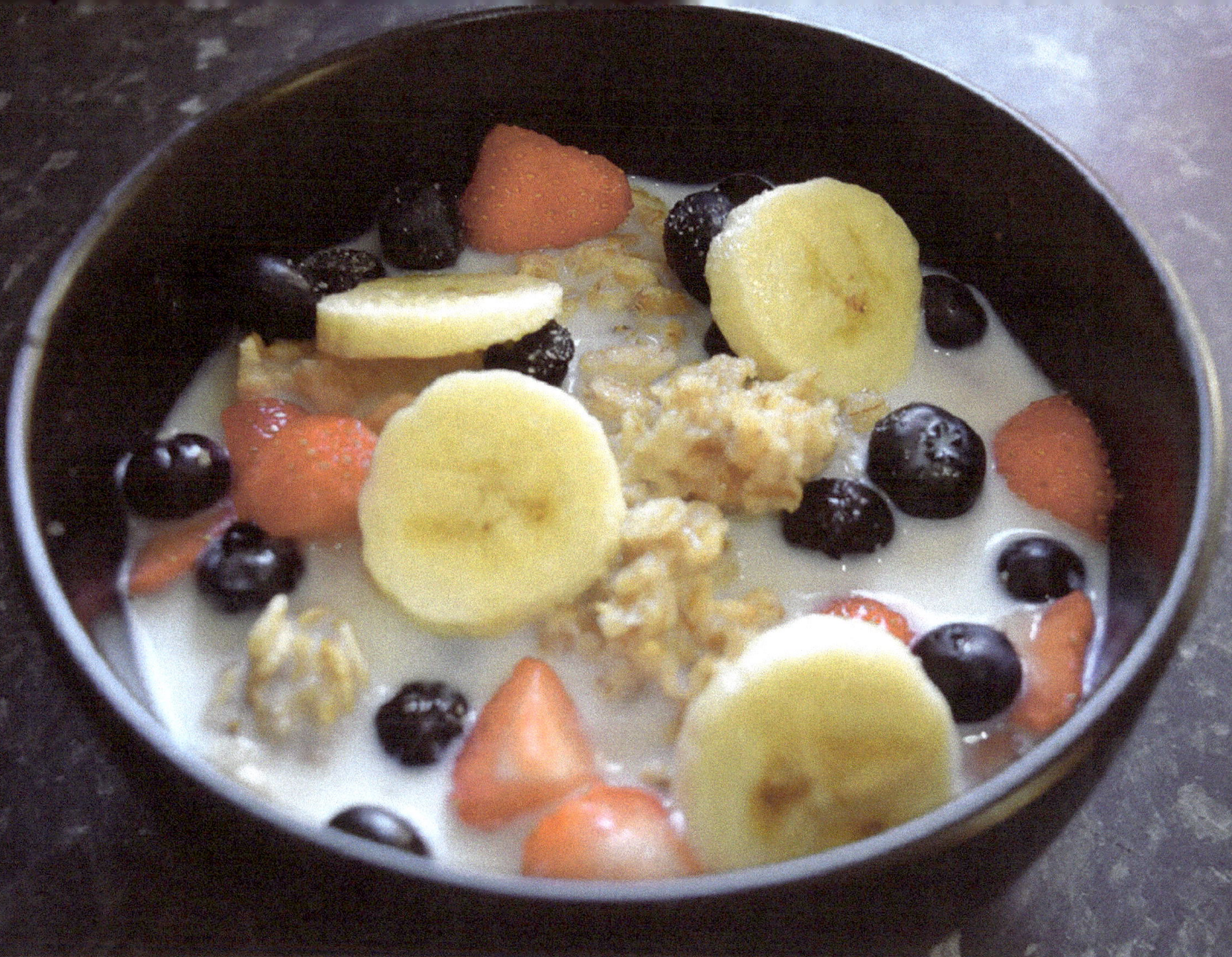

Fruit Porridge

Ingredients

- 35g porridge oats (cooked oatmeal)
- 150ml skimmed milk (1% milk)
- 2 tbsp. fat free natural yogurt (unflavored yogurt)
- A handful of frozen berries, defrosted

Method

1. Make up the porridge (cooked oatmeal) as per the packet instructions, using the skimmed milk.

2. Once it's been warmed up, top it with the yogurt (unflavored yogurt), berries and one level tsp. of runny honey.

3. You can add as much fruit as you like; there is no set rule for this meal. I love my fruit so I always put loads of fruit in. It's a very healthy and tasty breakfast. A great start for your day.

A little tip: add much more fat free natural yogurt (unflavored yogurt). I think it makes this breakfast taste so much better.

This is a great healthy breakfast. You can add as many fruits as you like. It all comes down to personal taste.

Ham and Egg Muffins

Ingredients

- 150g small mushrooms
- 60g smoked lean ham
- 2 spring onions
- low calorie cooking spray
- 4 large eggs
- 25ml skimmed milk (1% milk)
- salt and pepper

Method

1. Preheat the oven to Gas Mark 5 – 375f. Prepare your ingredients: quarter the mushrooms; dice the ham; trim and finely chop the spring onions.
2. Spray a non-stick frying pan with low calorie cooking spray and cook the mushrooms for ten minutes until golden. Mix the mushrooms, ham and onion together. Whisk the eggs and skimmed milk together and season to taste.
3. Line a muffin tin with paper cases. Spoon the mushroom mixture evenly between the cases and pour in the beaten egg. Bake in the oven for twenty to twenty-five minutes, or until slightly risen and golden. Leave to cool slightly for a few minutes before removing from the cases. Serve with baked beans, tomatoes and mushrooms.

Ham and egg muffins can be a great afternoon snack if you want. Or you can add other foods to make a meal of it. In this particular snack I added mushrooms. You can add onions, peppers or more if you prefer.

Like many of my meals they are not set in stone. You can add or take away many ingredients. It all comes down to personal taste. As long as you use natural ingredients it remains healthy and you can lose weight.

There are 6 breakfasts there, but you can get the idea from those breakfasts to change them slightly into a breakfast that you would like. Each person is different and we all like our food slightly differently. However from these listed above you can change them to suit your personal needs.

This dramatically changed the way I was eating because the way I was eating made me very overweight. So change was needed.

During the day I would just buy lots of fruit. Now I actually really like fruit so it wasn't a chore for me to buy and eat fruit. I'd eat apples, pears, oranges, bananas, grapes, strawberries, raspberries, and blueberries almost every single day. Eating fruit is obviously healthy and it actually kept me full.

I'm a taxi driver and normally I'd pull into a garage and grab a sandwich, chocolate bar and a bag of crisps (potato chips). I'd do this every day. So eating fruit is obviously much healthier and it's a lifestyle change.

In the evening I would have a meal. It's much healthier to cook your own meals. Generally cooking your own meals makes them free from excess fat and healthy. You can add spices, herbs and a homemade sauce to liven up any meal.

Generally when you cook a meal you would use a piece of meat. Any meat is good for you, providing you cut off the excess fat. The fat is not needed and it is no good for you. With the meat you would generally add vegetables or salad. This obviously is good for you. You can add plain couscous, rice or pasta to your meal. So you can see already that you can use many different ingredients to make your meal taste better. After all we all want that, a good tasting and filling meal. If it's healthy as well, all the better.

And of course you can add herbs and spices to the ingredients or add a homemade sauce.

Let me give you a few meals that I started off with. When I first started on my weight loss journey I wanted to keep everything as simple as possible.

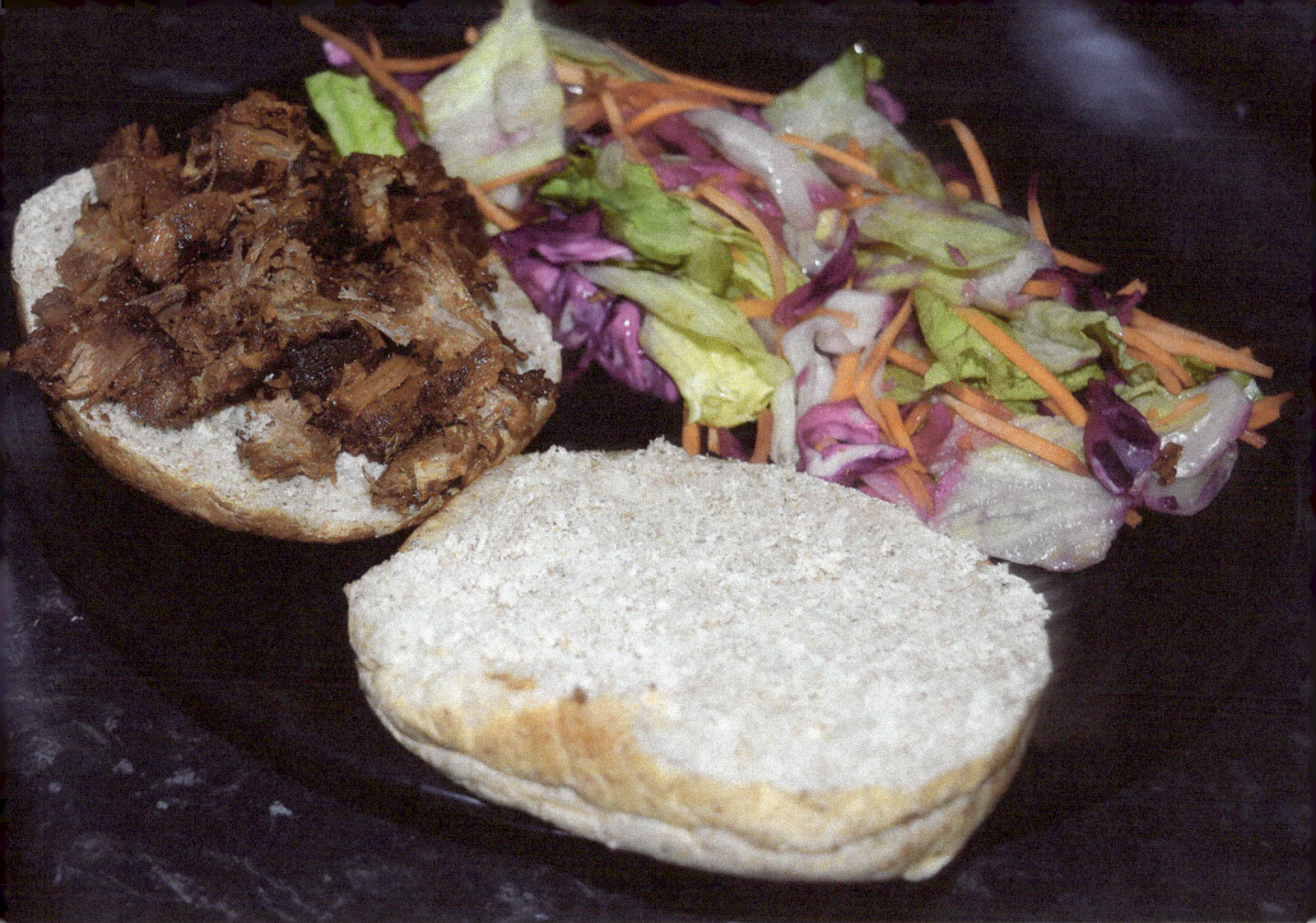

BBQ Pulled Pork

Ingredients

- 1.5-2kg pork shoulder, all fat removed
- 5 tbsp. worcester sauce (bold steak sauce)
- 1 tsp. mustard powder
- 500g passata (tomato sauce)
- 3 tbsp. balsamic vinegar (balsamic nectar)
- 2 cloves of garlic, crushed
- 3 tbsp. Canderel (Splenda)
- salt and freshly ground black pepper

Method

1. In a small bowl, mix passata (tomato sauce), Worcester sauce, balsamic vinegar, mustard powder, garlic, Canderel (Splenda) and seasoning. Transfer to a small pan and simmer for fifteen minutes, or until the sauce thickens.
2. Meanwhile, trim and remove all visible fat from the pork and sear all sides in a hot frying pan. Transfer to a slow cooker coat with the sauce and cook for eight to twelve hours on low.
3. Remove the pork from the slow cooker and place on a cutting board. Allow the meat to cool for approximately fifteen minutes, then shred into bite-sized pieces using two forks.
4. Remove the sauce from the pan and set aside to drizzle on the meat later.

This is an amazing meal, and very, very tasty. Homemade sauce primarily made from passata (tomato sauce) is excellent for making homemade sauces.

You can add a crisp salad, vegetables or maybe baked beans and homemade chips (French fries) to this.

This is one of my favorite meals.

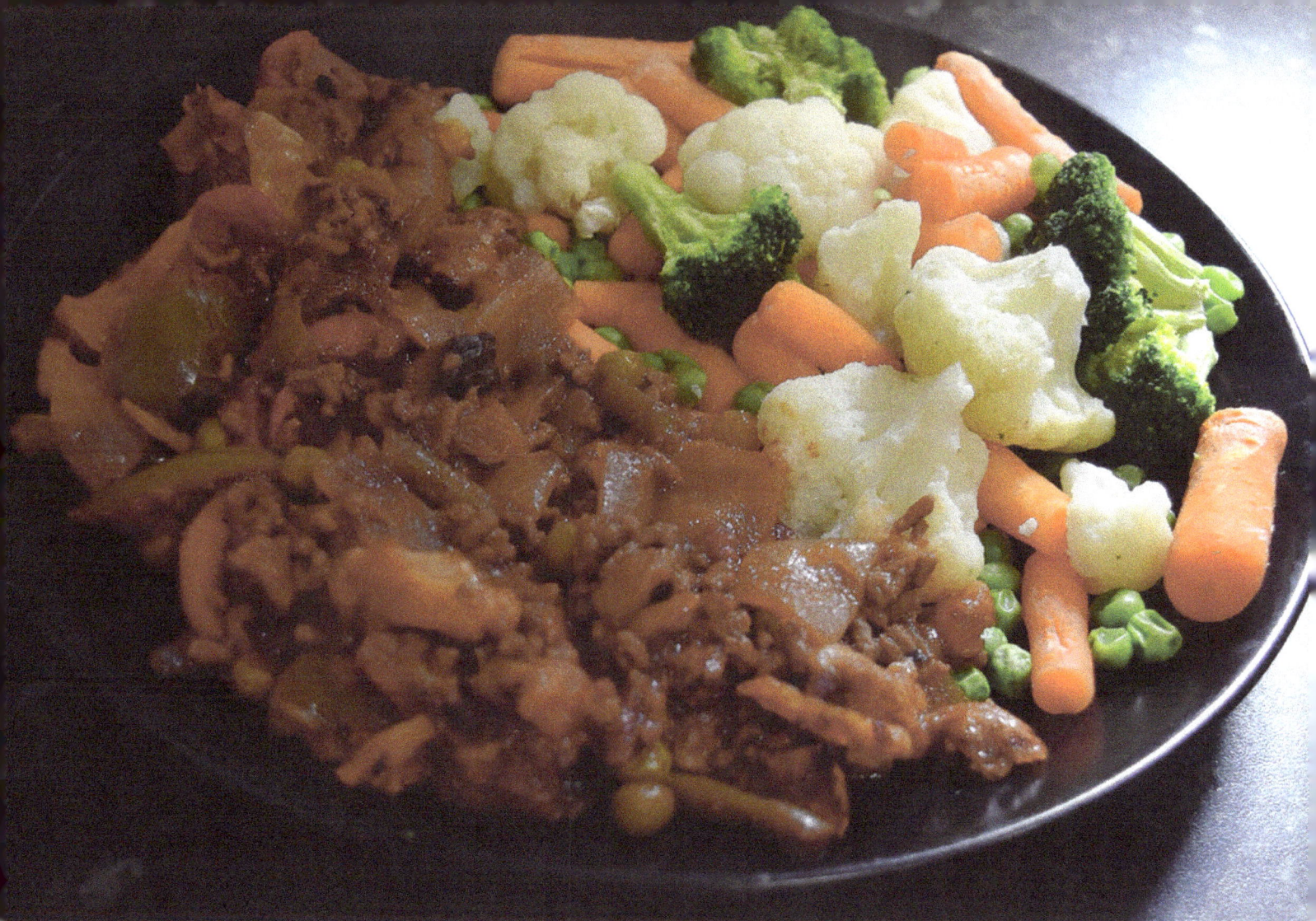

Bolognese Pasta Bake

Ingredients

- 250g dried pasta shapes
- 1 onion, finely chopped
- 2 celery sticks, finely chopped
- 1 carrot, finely chopped
- 250g mushrooms, chopped
- 3 garlic cloves
- 500g passata (tomato sauce)
- tin of chopped tomatos
- 3 tbsp worcester sauce (bold steak sauce)
- 500g extra lean mince 5% fat (ground beef)
- 250 ml beef stock

- 1 tsp. dried oregano
- 180g mozzarella, sliced
- low calorie cooking spray

Method

1. Cook pasta to packet instructions.
2. Fry the onion with low calorie cooking spray, celery, carrot, garlic, mushrooms and minced beef (ground beef) on a high heat for six to seven minutes
3. Add tomatoes/passata (tomato sauce), stock and oregano and cook over a medium heat for twenty minutes.
4. Mix the pasta in with the mince mixture and spoon into a casserole dish.
5. Top with the slices of mozzarella and baked in the oven for twenty-five to thirty minutes

Pasta is also another great food source to use and have in your meals. It's healthy and has carbohydrates for the energy you need.

With this meal I just added lots of veg to the meal. It's healthy and helps fill the plate up.

Cajun Chicken With Potato Wedges

Ingredients

- 4 chicken drumsticks, skinned
- 4 chicken thighs, skinned
- 900g large new potatoes, quartered into wedges
- 30g sachet Schwartz flavorful Cajun chicken recipe mix
- 8 mini corn on the cobs
- a handful of fresh flat-leaf parsley, chopped, to garnish

For the coleslaw:

- 200g summer cabbage, quartered, cored and shredded
- 2 carrots, coarsely grated
- salt
- 4 level tbsp. extra-light mayonnaise
- 4 spring onions, finely shredded

Method

1. Preheat your oven Gas Mark 6 – 400f. Cut a few slits into the chicken drumsticks and thighs and put them in a large roasting tin with the wedges. Sprinkle over the Cajun seasoning and toss everything together.
2. Roast in the oven for fifty minutes, mixing occasionally. Add the corn cobs halfway through the cooking time.
3. For the coleslaw, put the cabbage in a colander. Pour over a kettle full of just-boiled water, letting it drain, to soften the cabbage slightly. Cool it quickly with cold water and let it drain again.
4. Add the carrot to the colander. Sprinkle over a good pinch of salt and mix well (this both seasons the vegetables and draws out some of the moisture). Leave to drain for fifteen minutes. Transfer to a large bowl and mix together well with the mayonnaise and shredded spring onions.

5. Divide the spicy chicken, potatoes and corn cobs between four plates, garnish with chopped flat-leaf parsley and serve with the coleslaw on the side.

Using homemade chips (French fries) or wedges is fantastic. They are very healthy, taste great and can make most meals so much better to have.

Chili Beef & Vegetable Stir Fry

Ingredients

- 1 red chili pepper, deseeded & finely chopped
- bunch of spring onions
- 3cm ginger, peeled and grated
- 4 garlic cloves
- 300g of medium noodles
- 500g lean beef mince 5% fat (ground beef)
- 400g mixed stir fry vegetables
- 2 tbsp. light soy sauce (kikkoman)
- 2 tbsp. dark soy sauce (kikkoman)
- low calorie cooking spray

Method

1. Spray wok with low calorie cooking spray and put in the garlic, ginger and chili pepper and fry for a few minutes. Add all the beef mince (ground beef) and fry until cooked.
2. Then add stir fry vegetables and noodles. Keep cooking until the vegetables are tender. Add the soy sauce and fry for one minute.

With this meal you can add as many vegetables as you like. It's a very versatile meal.

Chicken Tikka Masala

Without question, chicken tikka masala is a brilliant curry that makes people very happy. Of course it's inspired by fantastic Indian cooking, but is in fact an Anglo-Indian evolution, created to suit British palates. When you make it, you'll be super proud. You can use top-quality chicken, it's loads of fun to marinate and grill, the method rocks, and it's highly unlikely you'll find a better expression. I love to make my own paratha breads to serve with it too—check out the recipe at the bottom of the page. Dig a hole in the garden and get grilling!

Ingredients

- 1 level tsp. ground cloves
- 1 level tsp. ground cumin
- 2 heaped tsp. sweet smoked paprika
- 2 heaped tsp. garam masala
- 3 lemons
- 6 cloves of garlic
- 1 thumb-sized piece of ginger
- 6 heaped tbsp. natural yogurt (unflavored yogurt)
- 800g skinless boneless chicken breasts
- 3 fresh green or yellow chili peppers

For the sauce:

- 2 onions
- 4 cloves of garlic
- 1–2 fresh red chili peppers
- 30 g fresh coriander
- low calorie cooking spray
- 1 level tablespoon ground coriander
- 2 level teaspoons turmeric
- 6 tbsp ground almonds
- 2 x 400g tins of plum tomatoes

- 1 chicken stock cube
- 2 x 400g tins of light coconut milk

For the paratha breads (optional):

- 300g wholegrain bread flour
- 300g plain flour

Method

1. Put the cloves, cumin and one heaped teaspoon each of paprika and garam masala into a small pan and toast for one minute to bring them back to life. Then tip into a large bowl. Finely grate in the zest of one lemon, squeeze in all its juice, crush in the garlic, peel and finely grate in the ginger, and add the yogurt and one teaspoon of sea salt. Cut the chicken breasts into 5cm chunks, and then massage all that flavor into the meat. Skewer up the chicken chunks, interspersing them with lemon wedges and chunks of green or yellow chili pepper, but don't squash them together too much. Place on a tray, cover with Clingfilm and marinate in the fridge for at least two hours, but preferably overnight.

2. For the sauce, peel the onions and garlic, and then finely slice with the red chili peppers and coriander stalks (reserving the leaves for later). Put it all into a large casserole pan on a medium-high heat with a low calorie cooking spray and cook for around twenty minutes, or until golden, stirring regularly. Add the ground coriander, turmeric and remaining one heaped tsp. each of paprika and garam masala. Cook for two minutes, then add and toast the almonds. Pour in the tomatoes, crumble in the stock cube and add 300ml of boiling water. Simmer for five minutes, and then stir in the coconut milk. Simmer for a final forty minutes, stirring occasionally, then season to perfection.

3. When you're ready to cook the chicken, drizzle it with a low calorie cooking spray, then grill on a hot barbecue, in a screaming hot griddle pan or under a hot grill, turning until it's very golden and gnarly on all sides. Slice the chicken off the skewers straight into the sauce, reserving the lemons. Simmer for two minutes while you use tongs to squeeze some jammy lemons over the curry to taste. Swirl through some more yogurt, sprinkle with the coriander leaves, and serve with parathas or fluffy basmati rice.

Cooking curries is one of my favorite meals. You can still fry all the vegetables but use low calorie cooking spray instead of olive oil. There are dozens of different tasting and strength curries you can cook. All are healthy and great tasting.

Curries are the most varied meal you will ever cook. You can make them very mild (korma) or have them very hot (vindaloo) or you can use different mustards to make it spicier. The amount of varieties of curries is in the hundreds.

It's not how much you eat, but what you eat that matters.

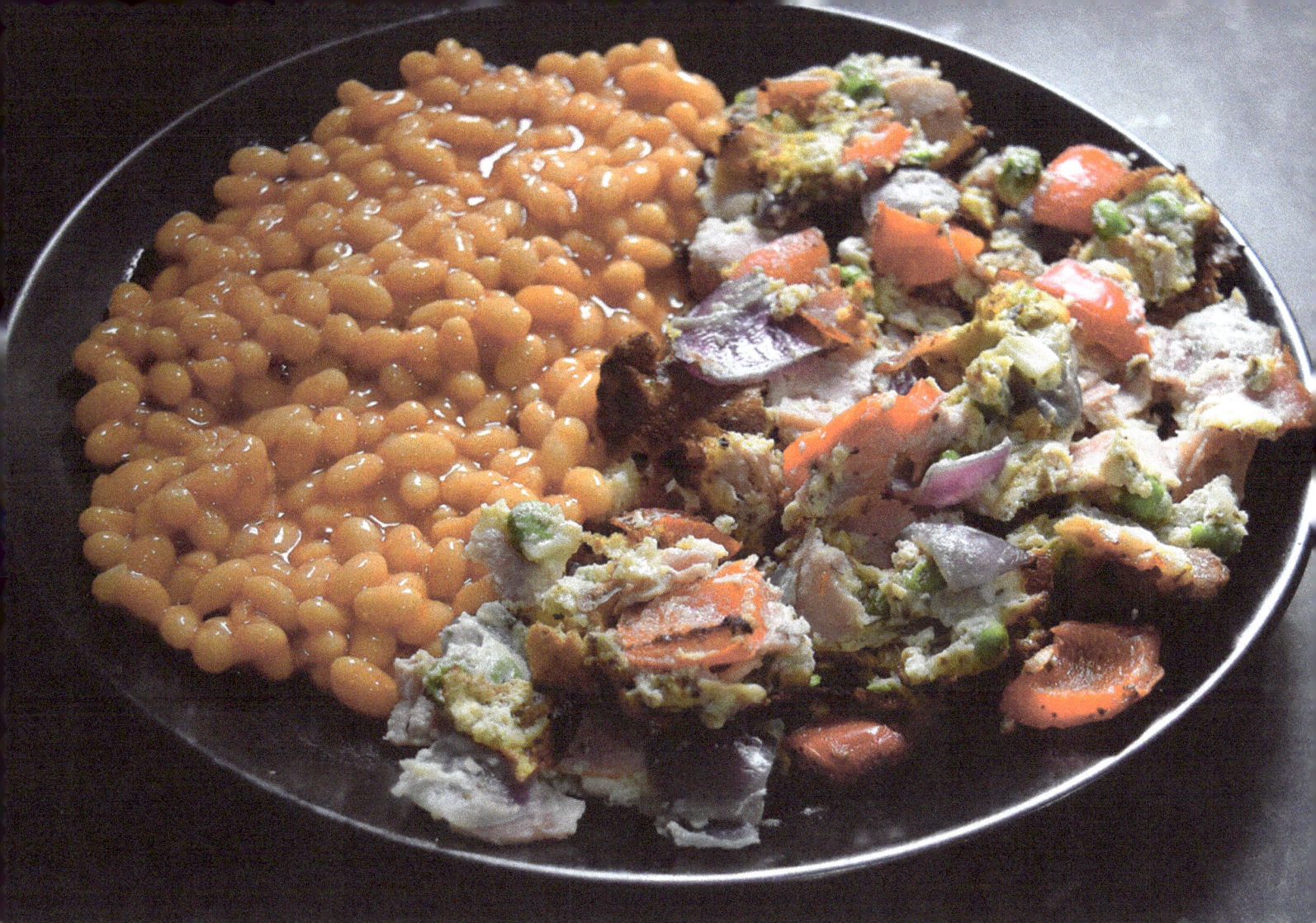

Frittata

Ingredients

- 50g frozen peas
- 4 eggs
- 1 red onion, roughly chopped
- 1 red pepper, cubed
- A small handful of fresh mint, shredded
- low calorie cooking spray
- 100g lean ham, diced

Method

1. Boil 50g frozen peas for three to four minutes, then drain. Preheat your grill to high.

2. Crack four eggs into a medium bowl and beat well. Stir in one roughly chopped red onion, one cubed red pepper, a small handful of shredded fresh mint and the peas, and season well.

3. Spray a medium ovenproof frying pan with low calorie cooking spray and place over a medium heat. Pour in the egg mixture and cook for four to five minutes, or until the base is set.

4. Cube the 100g canned lean ham, scatter over the frittata, then grill for four to five minutes, or until set and the top is bubbling and slightly golden. Allow to cool completely, and then cut into six wedges and divide between two lunchboxes. Chill until ready to eat.

Creamy Pasta Bake

Ingredients

- 250g dried penne pasta
- 3 courgettes
- 1 red and 1 yellow pepper
- 2 red onions
- 4 garlic cloves
- low calorie cooking spray
- 2 x 400g cans chopped tomatoes
- 2 tsp. dried mixed herbs
- salt and freshly ground black pepper
- 300g fat free natural yogurt (unflavored yogurt)

Method

1. Preheat the oven to Gas Mark 6 - 400f.
2. Cook the penne according to the packet instructions, drain and set aside.
3. Cut the courgettes into thick strips, deseed and cut the peppers into strips, peel and roughly chop the onions and peel and finely chop the garlic. Place the vegetables in a large roasting tin and sprinkle over the garlic. Spray lightly with low calorie cooking spray and bake in the oven for fifteen to twenty minutes or until tender.
4. When cooked, transfer the vegetables to a bowl. Add the chopped tomatoes and dried herbs, season well and stir to combine. Place the mixture in an oven proof dish.
5. Beat the natural yogurt (unflavored yogurt) until smooth, season and toss with the drained pasta. Spoon over the vegetables and return to the oven to cook for a further fifteen to twenty minutes. Remove from the oven, divide between four warmed serving plates, and serve immediately with some boiled green beans.

Tip: When cooked this dish can be frozen for up to one month.

There are six meals to get you started. However you can make normal meals as well, like ham, egg and chips.

Homemade chips (French fries) are a real winner. Cut a potato into chips. Spray with low calorie cooking spray and put into the oven at Gas Mark 6 – 400f for thirty-five to forty minutes. Then you have tasty healthy chips.

Don't forget, you can add any spices, herbs or homemade sauces to your meals to make them livelier.

The key to successfully losing weight is to make your meals filling, tasty and healthy. The longer you do this, the more adept you become at making any meal for any time of the day.

This Book Is Not a Diet Book; It's a Lifestyle Change Book

It didn't take me long to work out that this lifestyle change was a lot easier than I first thought to go from eating the way I did eating takeaways (takeouts) and ready made meals to cooking my own food. I used to buy most my meals premade in packets or buy takeaway (takeout). There is so much added to packet food, stuff you don't want or need.

To cook yourself a meal is very healthy and you know exactly what has gone into the meal. You can make the meal as spicy as you like, or just add a plain homemade sauce to liven your meal up.

You can add any amount of spices or herbs and you will transform any meal. You can also add soy sauce, Worcester or balsamic vinegar sauce to add taste. Or mix up a homemade sauce.

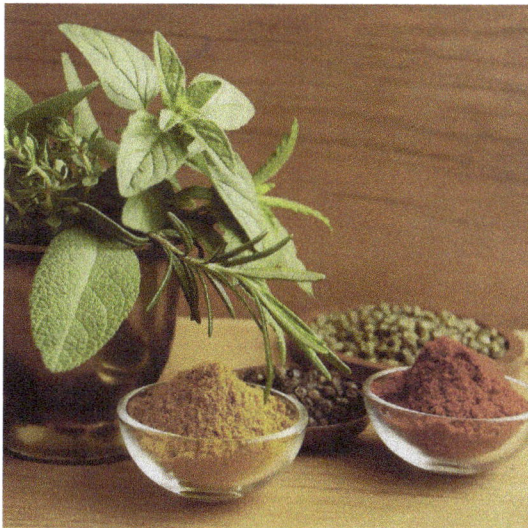

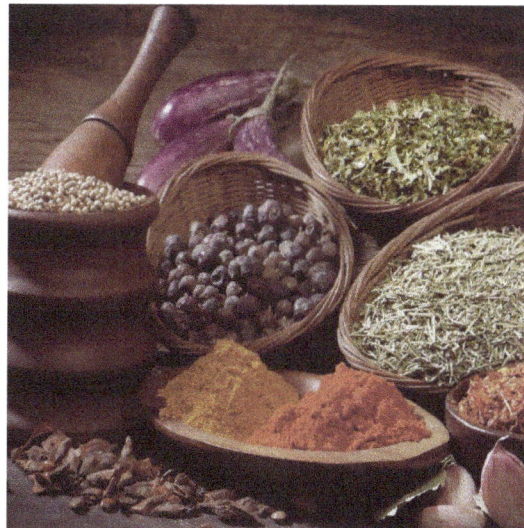

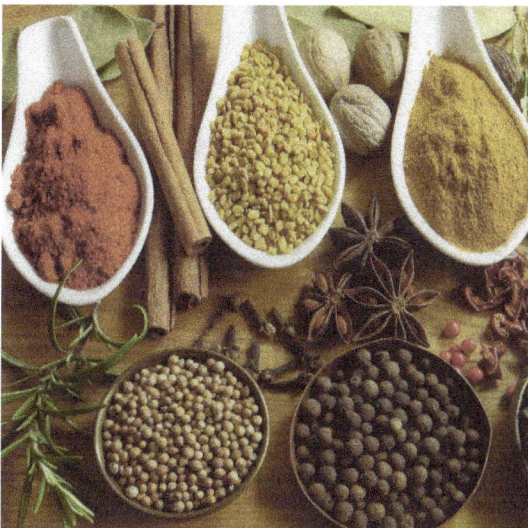

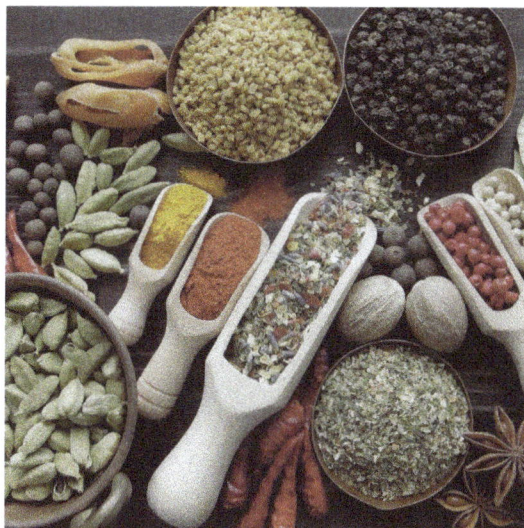

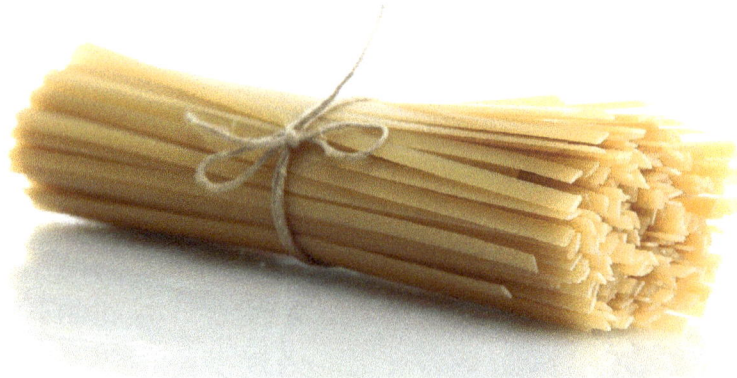

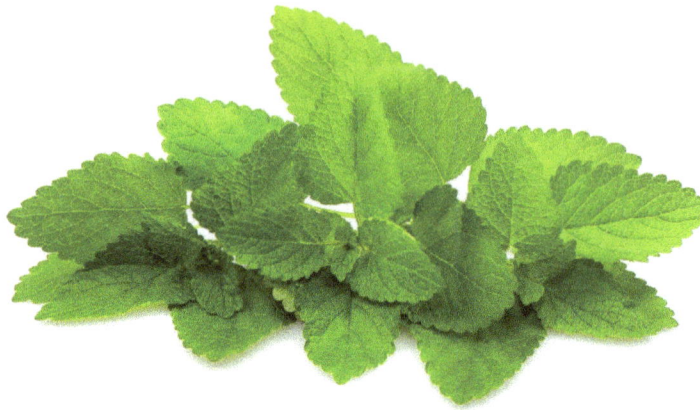

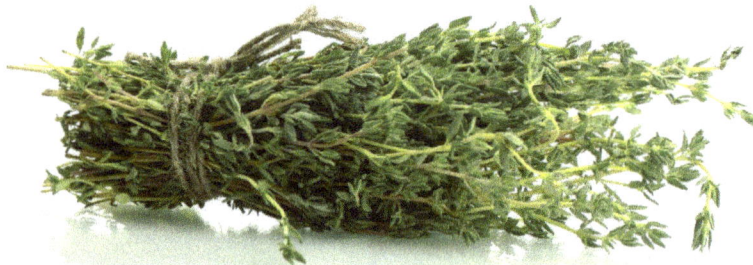

Two good things to use as a homemade sauce are: an ordinary tin of chopped tomatoes, add a couple of spices or herbs, soy sauce, Worcester sauce, balsamic vinegar, garlic ginger parsley, thyme, or salt and pepper. This is the basis of any sauce; you can also add peppers, mushrooms and onions. This makes a very good filling sauce to go with any meal.

The other thing to use is passata (tomato sauce). This is a tomato based sauce. It comes in a few different flavors. I add Worcester sauce, chicken stock 500ml and herbs to it to make a nice tasting sauce.

The whole idea is to cook your own food and to make it as tasty as possible; every person on earth wants their meal to be filling and to be tasty, but you're making it healthy as well.

This Simple Change to Your Way of Eating Will Benefit You Very Quickly

We are all different as people. Some of us need support, help, and guidance. Some of us can do this alone. The whole idea of this book is to give you a way into a lifestyle change. Now how you go about that change is totally personal, but use this book as a guideline into your new way of thinking.

After a short time you will notice a change. A drop in clothes size for example. You are more lithe and able to move about easier. Use these changes as motivation to carry on. Soon you will notice a very big difference. You may even ask yourself why you didn't do this earlier.

Please, keep a pair of trousers and a shirt you wear now. Keep them to one side so in a month or so you can try them on and you will see the visible difference. For me personally there is no better feeling than putting on the jeans I used to wear. I don't need anyone to tell me I've lost weight, I can physically see it.

There is an old adage, a very true adage: you are what you eat. After a while of cooking your own meals and you see the weight drop off, you begin to understand that adage very clearly.

If you're like I was, you are a lazy eater. You would buy packet meals or get takeaways (takeouts). This is lazy eating and it's incredibly unhealthy. Learn to cook for yourself and immediately you become a much healthier person. Trust me, it won't take you long to visibly see the difference in yourself.

Okay, it's possible you may not be a good cook, but if you can learn to cook even a simple meal it's a great start. You might be better off going to cookery lessons as opposed to joining a slimming club. Cooking for yourself is the key to eating healthier and losing weight.

Chapter Three

Stage Two

After two months I had lost 3 Stone in weight (42 pounds). The clothes I needed to wear were now smaller than what I used to wear, so I was very happy with my progress but I thought to myself, I needed to keep changing my food plans. I didn't want my body getting used to the food. I wanted to carry on losing weight. I still had a long way to go to achieve my target of losing all my excess weight in a year.

I had never had a breakfast before in my life. Now for the last two months I've been having a breakfast every day and I had lost 3 Stone (42 pounds). I was amazed. I was actually eating more but losing weight. Just goes to show, it's not how much you eat but it's what you eat that matters.

I had lost 3 Stone (42 pounds) and I wanted to lose all my excess weight. The big trouble for me was that I had no idea how much weight I needed to lose in total. This is another thing that has become clear to me now. It's not how much you weigh that matters; it's how you feel inside. Every person you meet will have an opinion on how much you should weigh. Just nod, say yes and agree. It's how you feel inside that really matters.

So I thought, okay how can I change? So after some thought I decided to have a lunch as well as a breakfast. So I cut down a lot on the fruit I was eating and made a certain time of the day I would eat a lunch.

I searched the internet for ideas on lunch. I had never had a lunch in my life, and never really thought about it to be honest.

Here are the lunches I made myself.

Bacon And Mushroom Quiche

Ingredients

- low calorie cooking spray
- 220g bacon, cut into 1cm pieces
- 110g mushrooms, sliced
- 2 cloves garlic
- 3 large eggs
- 150g fat free cottage cheese
- 3–4 cherry tomatoes, halved
- 2 tbsp. fresh chopped parsley
- 80g reduced fat cheddar
- salt and freshly ground black pepper

Method

1. Remove all visible fat from the bacon and fry with low calorie cooking spray for a few minutes. Add the mushrooms and garlic, season well and continue to cook for four to five minutes, and then set aside.
2. Preheat the oven to Gas Mark 5 – 375f.
3. Spoon the bacon mixture into a flan dish.
4. Mix the eggs, cottage cheese, parsley and cheddar cheese in a bowl and spoon over the bacon mixture.
5. Top with the tomato halves and bake at Gas Mark 5 – 375f for fifteen to twenty minutes until just set.

You can have this as a lunch or as an afternoon snack.

Bean Burgers

Ingredients

- 1 carrot, chopped
- 100g potato, peeled and chopped
- 1 red onion, finely chopped
- 1 red chili pepper, deseeded and finely chopped
- 100g canned mixed beans, drained and rinsed
- 60g canned green lentils, drained and rinsed
- 1 egg
- 2 tsp. ground cumin
- 1 tsp. ground cinnamon
- 4 tbsp. finely chopped coriander leaves
- salt and freshly ground black pepper
- low calorie cooking spray

Method

1. Place all the ingredients in a food processor, season well and blend until well combined. Transfer to a bowl and chill for three to four hours or overnight.
2. Preheat the oven to Gas Mark 5 – 375f. Divide the bean mixture into two portions and shape each into a burger. Place on a baking tray lined with baking parchment, spray with low calorie cooking spray and cook for twelve to fifteen minutes or until golden.

Bean burgers are great with a tin of beans and homemade chips (French fries). Or you can have them with a crisp salad.

BLT And Pepper Sandwich

Ingredients

- 1 yellow pepper, halved and deseeded
- 2 lean bacon rashers, all visible fat removed
- 1 level tbsp. extra-light mayonnaise
- 1 tbsp. fat free natural yogurt (unflavored yogurt)
- Shredded iceberg lettuce
- 1 small tomato, sliced
- 2 slices 400g wholegrain bread

Method

1. Preheat the grill to hot. Grill the pepper halves for ten minutes, then transfer to a sealable plastic bag and set aside to cool for ten minutes.
2. Meanwhile, grill the bacon on both sides until cooked to your liking. Cut into large pieces and set aside.
3. Mix the mayonnaise and natural yogurt (unflavored yogurt) then spread on a slice of toast or bread. Add the lettuce, tomato and bacon. Peel off and discard the pepper skin and add the flesh to the sandwich, topping with another slice of toast or bread.

Chicken And Tomato Soup

Ingredients

- 1 onion, peeled and finely chopped
- 2 carrots, peeled and grated
- 2 lean back bacon rashers, all visible fat removed, finely chopped
- 2 large skinless and boneless chicken breasts, cut into thin strips
- 600g tined chopped tomatoes
- 400ml chicken stock
- 1 tbsp. chopped rosemary
- finely grated zest and juice of 1 lemon
- salt and freshly ground black pepper
- chopped fresh flat-leaf parsley, to garnish

Method

1. Place the onion, carrots and bacon in a large non-stick saucepan and stir-fry for two to three minutes.
2. Add the chicken, tomatoes, stock, rosemary and lemon zest and juice. Bring to the boil, stir, then cover and simmer on a medium heat for fifteen minutes, stirring occasionally. Season to taste and serve sprinkled with chopped parsley.

Buy yourself a soup maker. There are loads of homemade soups you can make. You can make a soup out of anything really. So get your creative head on.

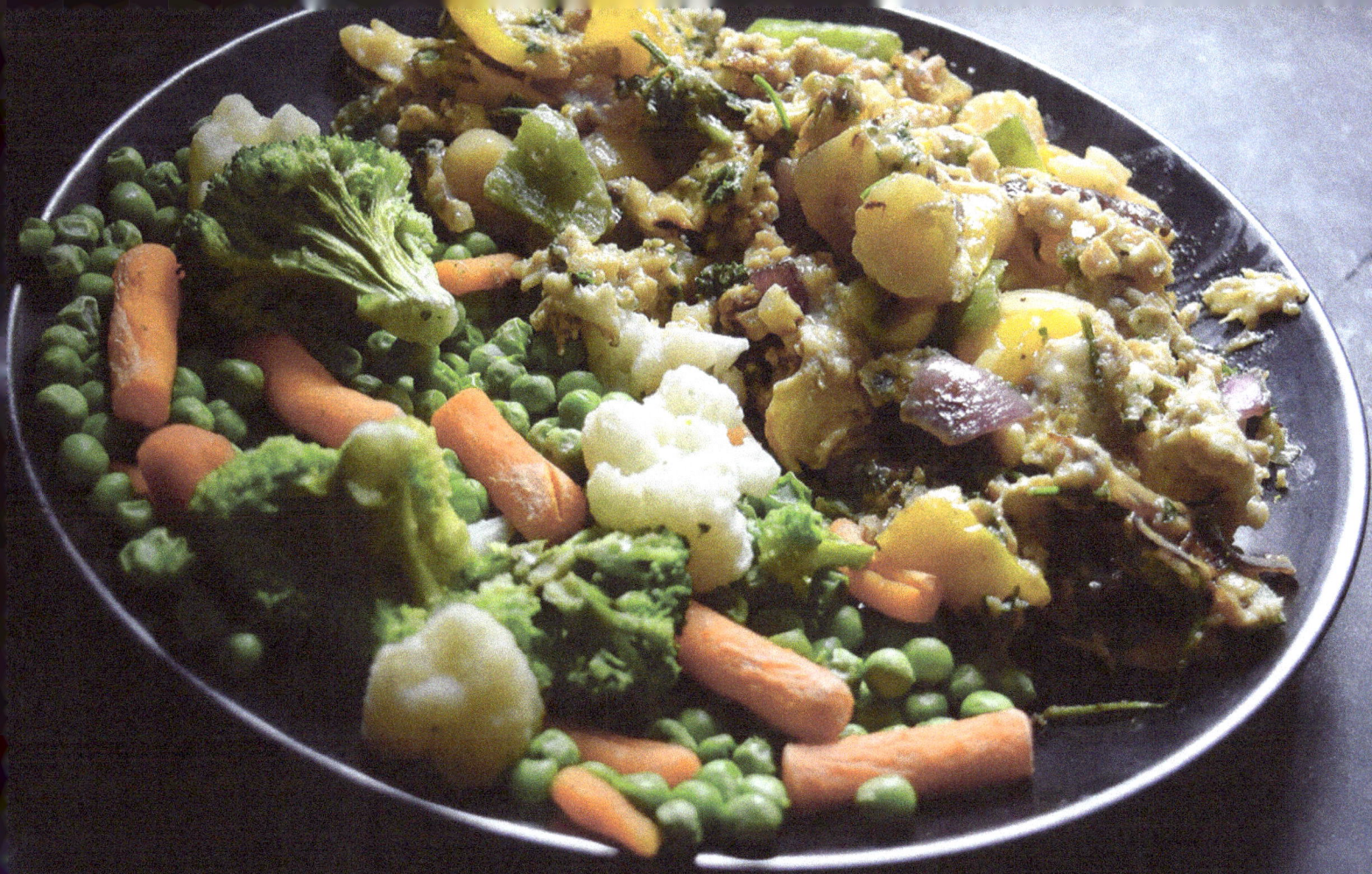

Spanish Omelette

Ingredients

- 1 medium onion, thinly sliced
- 275ml of vegetable stock
- 175g small new potatoes
- 5 large eggs
- salt and pepper
- 1 tbsp. finely chopped parsley
- low calorie cooking spray

Method

1. Put the onion and stock in a heavy saucepan, cover with a lid and bring to boil. Boil for five minutes, then uncover the pan and simmer gently over a low heat for about twenty-five minutes, until the onions are tender and golden and all the liquid has been absorbed. Strain off any liquid that has not evaporated.

2. Meanwhile, cook the potatoes in lightly salted boiling water until tender. Drain, remove the skins and slice thinly into rounds.

3. Break the eggs into a bowl and beat lightly with a fork. Add some salt and pepper, and then stir in the cooked onion and potatoes and the chopped parsley.

4. Heat a seasoned or non-stick 20cm frying pan and spray the base and sides with low calorie cooking spray. Pour the egg mixture into the hot pan and reduce the heat to a bare simmer. Cook very gently over the lowest possible heat for about fifteen minutes, or until the underneath is set but the top is still slightly runny.

5. Place the pan under a preheated hot grill, just long enough to set and lightly brown the top of the omelet. Slide the omelet out onto a serving plate. Cut into wedges and serve with a crisp salad.

You can have this meal with veg, salad, rice, pasta even a tin of baked beans. I had this meal all by itself. I added peppers and mushrooms to this meal. You can add as many vegetables as you like; it's one of those types of meals. Very filling and tasty and very healthy.

Egg Fried Rice

Ingredients

- low calorie cooking spray
- 350g cooked and cooled long-grain or jasmine/Thai fragrant rice
- 200g frozen peas
- salt and freshly ground black pepper
- 2 large eggs, lightly beaten
- 3 tbsp. light soy sauce (kikkoman)
- 400g fresh bean sprouts, rinsed
- 6 spring onions, very finely sliced

Method

1. Spray a wok or large frying pan with low calorie cooking spray and place over a high heat. When it is almost at smoking point, add the cooked rice and stir-fry for about three minutes.
2. Add the peas, stir-fry for five minutes and season well. Add the beaten eggs and stir-fry for another minute.
3. Stir in the soy sauce, bean sprouts and most of the spring onion and cook for two minutes or until the eggs have set.
4. Scatter over the remaining spring onions to serve.

I had this a few times. I added homemade curry sauce and homemade chips (French fries).

Mexican Chicken Fajitas

Ingredients

- 1 red pepper, halved, deseeded and finely sliced
- 1 green pepper, halved, deseeded and finely sliced
- 2 medium red onions, halved and finely sliced
- 2-3 skinless boneless chicken breasts, cut into chunks
- 1 tsp. smoked paprika
- 1 tsp. cumin
- 2 fresh red chili peppers, deseeded and finely chopped
- juice of 1 lime
- low calorie cooking spray
- salt and freshly ground black pepper
- For the salsa
- ½-1 fresh red chili pepper, deseeded and finely chopped
- 15 ripe cherry tomatoes, halved
- small handful of finely chopped coriander
- salt and freshly ground black pepper
- juice of 1 lime

Method

Put your griddle pan on a high heat. Halve and deseed your pepper and cut it into thin strips. Peel, halve, and finely slice your onion. Slice your chicken lengthways into long strips roughly the same size as your pepper strips.

Put the peppers, onion, and chicken into a bowl with the paprika and cumin. Squeeze over the juice of half a lime, drizzle over a lug of olive oil, season with a good pinch of pepper and mix well. Put to one side to marinate for 5 minutes or so while you make your salsa.

Finely chop your chilli. Roughly chop your tomatoes and the coriander, stalks and all. Put the chilli and tomatoes into a second bowl with the salt and pepper and the juice of 1 lime, then stir in your chopped coriander.

Use a pair of tongs to put all the pieces of pepper, onion, and chicken into your preheated pan to cook for 6 to 8 minutes until the chicken is golden and cooked through. As the pan will be really hot, keep turning the pieces of chicken and vegetables over so they don't burn – you just want them to lightly chargrill to give you a lovely flavour. Give the pan a little love and attention and you'll be laughing.

To make the guacamole, squeeze a handful of cherry tomatoes onto a board. Finely chop up the flesh with ½ -1 red chilli and a handful of coriander leaves, including the top part of the stalks.

At the table, carefully help yourselves to the chicken and vegetables straight from the hot grill pan. Just be sure to put it down on top of something that won't burn, like a chopping board. Serve with bowls of natural yogurt and guacamole alongside your Cheddar, a grater, and your lovely fresh salsa.

Sweet Chili Chicken

Ingredients

- 4 garlic cloves, crushed
- 110ml soy sauce (kikkoman)
- 2 tbsp. sweet chili sauce
- 2 tbsp. harissa powder (chili powder)
- 12 boneless and skinless chicken thighs
- salt and freshly ground black pepper
- a handful of fresh coriander, chopped

Method

1. Preheat your oven to gas mark 6 – 400f. Place the garlic, soy sauce, sweet chili sauce and harissa powder (chili powder) into a small bowl and mix. Pour over the chicken and toss together to coat evenly.
2. Place the chicken in a single layer on a non-stock baking tray. Season and bake for twenty-five to thirty minutes, or until cooked through
3. Remove the chicken from the oven, scatter over the coriander and serve with the lime juice squeezed over.

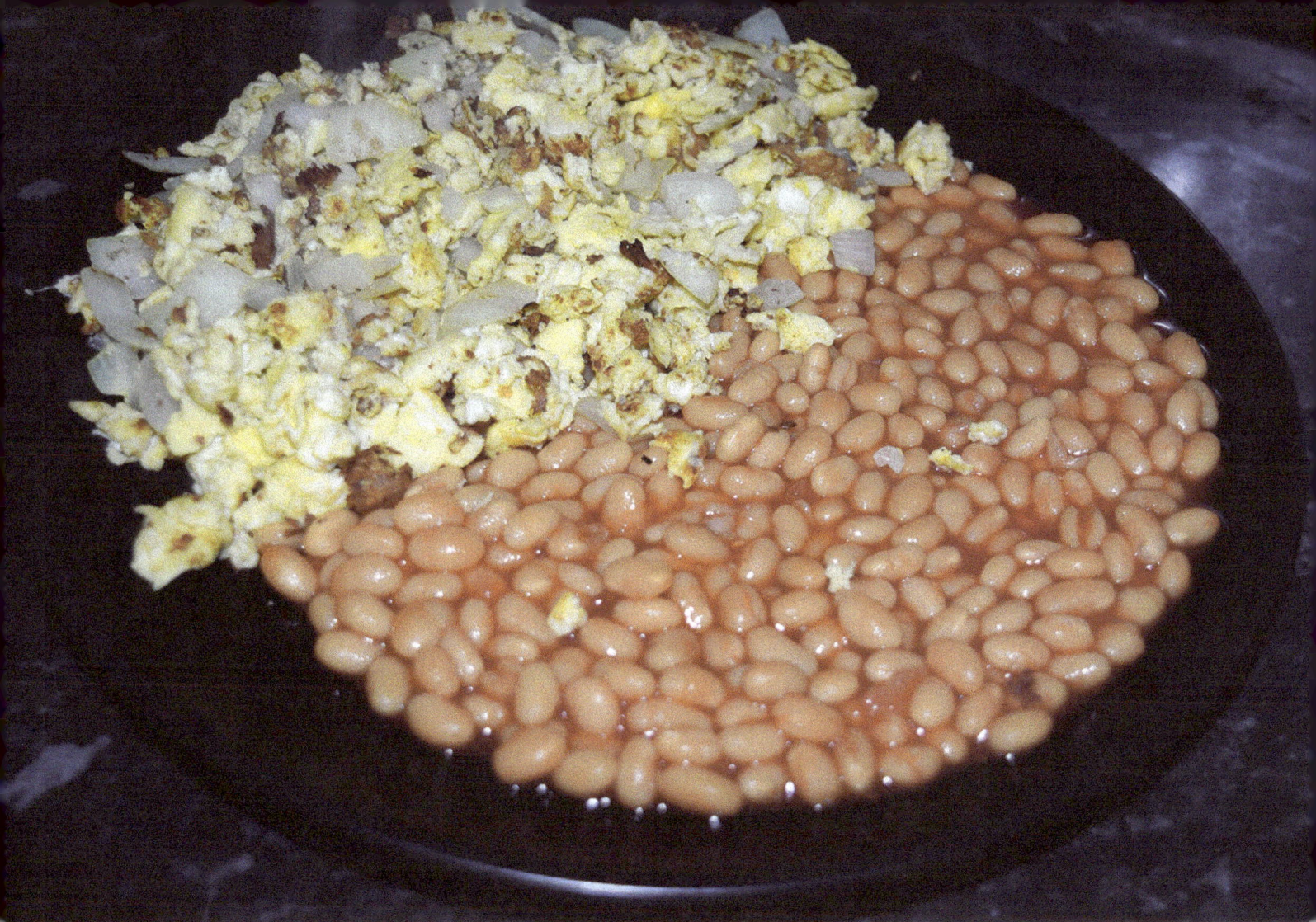

Omelette

Ingredients

- low calorie cooking spray
- 3 large eggs
- onion
- mushrooms
- salt and freshly ground black pepper

Method

1. Break the eggs into a bowl, season and a teaspoon of cold water. Beat gently with a fork to combine the whites and yolks. Do not overbeat or you will not end up with a fluffy light omelet.

2. Put the pan over a medium heat and spray the base and sides lightly with low calorie cooking spray. When the pan is really hot, pour in the eggs, tilting the pan to spread the omelette mixture evenly over the base.

3. When the underside of the omelette is set and golden and there is virtually no liquid egg left, fold the omelette over and slide it out of the pan to a warm plate and add your choice of fillings.

An omelette is a great food to eat. You can add any number of any other foods to make an omelette: onions, ham, bacon, mushrooms, cheese and peppers just to name a few.

An omelette is a great start to the day—a brilliant breakfast. I made this omelette with four eggs, onion and cheese. I had it with a tin of beans.

If you wanted you can have an omelette in the afternoon just as a snack. Eggs and beans are a good protein source with very few calories. So having an omelette as a breakfast or as a mid-afternoon snack is fine. You can still lose weight.

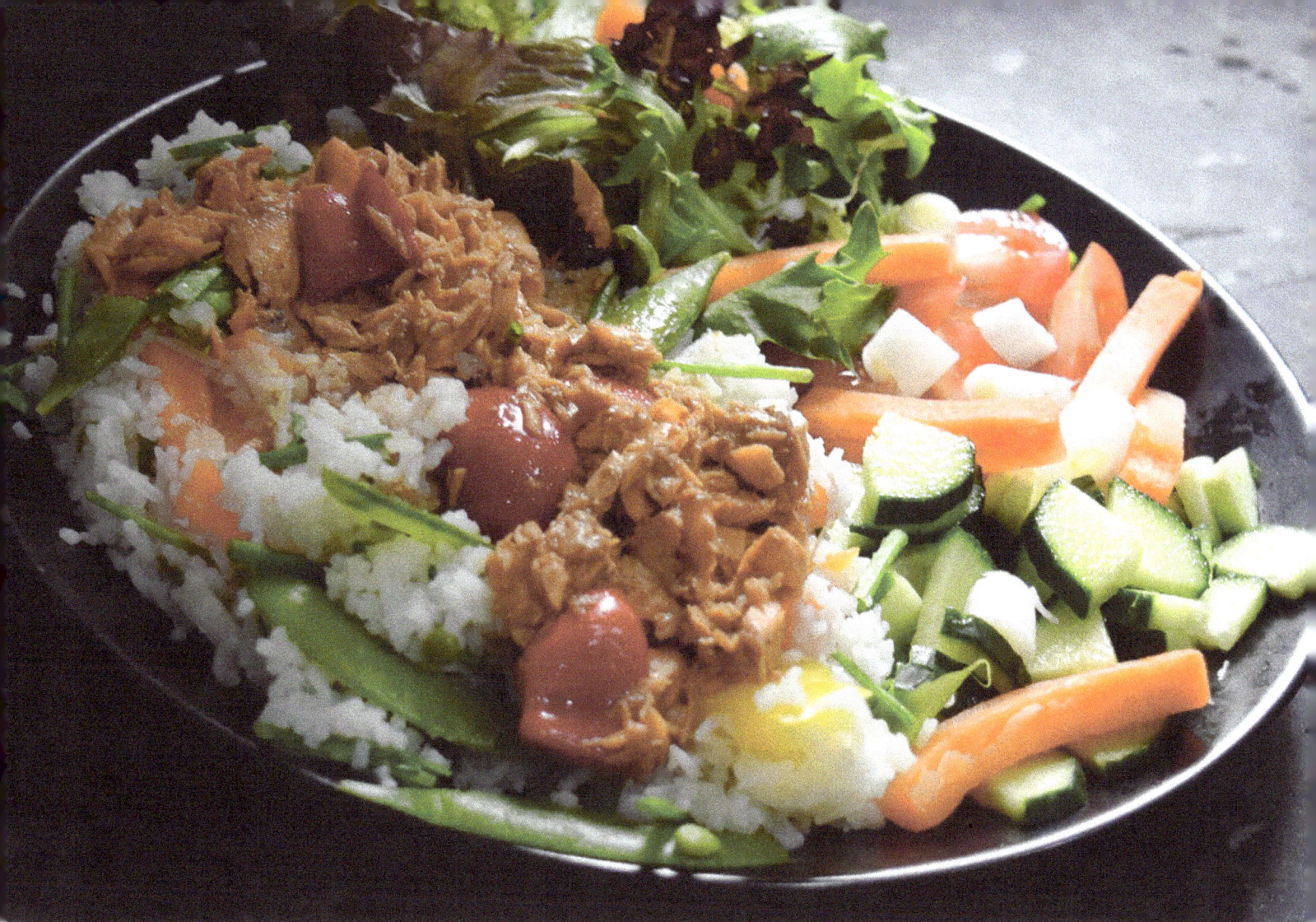

Salmon & Wild Rice

Ingredients

- 450g skinless salmon fillets
- 150g dried wholegrain basmati and wild rice
- 300g sugar snap peas
- 1 yellow pepper
- 2 carrots, peeled and cut into matchsticks
- 6 spring onions, trimmed and sliced
- 25g pack chives, finely snipped
- salt and freshly ground black pepper

For The dressing

- 5 tbsp. light soy sauce
- 1 tsp. peeled and grated root ginger
- 1 garlic clove, peeled and crushed
- 1 red chili pepper, deseeded and finely chopped
- 6 tbsp. lime juice
- 2 tbsp. canderel (splenda)

Method

1. Preheat the oven to Gas Mark 5 – 375f.
2. Place all the dressing ingredients in a clean jam jar. Cover and shake to mix well and set aside.
3. Season the salmon, place on a baking tray lined with non-stick baking parchment and bake for ten to twelve minutes or until just cooked.
4. Transfer the salmon to a snug-fitting shallow dish, pour over half of the dressing and set aside to cool. Flake the flesh into bite-sized pieces and set aside.
5. Meanwhile, bring a large saucepan of water to the boil, add the rice and simmer for twenty-five minutes, adding the sugar snap peas, yellow pepper and carrots for the last five minutes of cooking time.
6. Drain and cool under cold running water, then drain again.
7. Place the rice, sugar snap peas and carrots into a large bowl. Add the spring onions, chives and the remaining dressing and toss to mix well. Add the cooled salmon flakes and any dressing and mix gently. Season to taste before serving.

This is another meal you can do things with. You can add dills, or any other herbs and spices to make the rice wilder. You can make this a lot hotter if you prefer. Try cooking this with a Scotch Bonnet. You can add different vegetables if you like. It's a very tasty healthy meal.

You Are What You Eat

From these lunches and breakfast you will get a very good idea on how to make yourself a good, tasty, healthy meal. You will notice the ingredients and make a variety of anything you have seen in this book and come up with your own ideas. The list is endless to how many meals you can make yourself. Personally I had several more breakfasts not mentioned and about twenty more lunches I've not listed. I just wanted to give you an idea on the ingredients so you can make up your own meals, each person has their own foods they like or dislike.

I've said this before and I'll say it again. This is not a diet, it's a lifestyle change. You will benefit for it forever and live a longer healthier life. You just need to change your way of looking at food and how you eat.

I will say this though. Yes this is a lifestyle change, but I considered it a diet for the first year. It helped me to achieve my target by saying I was on a diet. However, the truth in the matter was that it was a lifestyle change because I'll carry on eating like this even when I've lost all my weight. So yes, it is a lifestyle change, but in the first year I told myself I was on a diet. We all have our own ways on making us do things. This was my way.

It's Not How Much You Eat; It's What You Eat That Matters

It's a fact. We all fancy a little treat now and again. I'm no different from all of you. But I would tell myself, no Tim, do not have a treat. It will slow your weight loss down. Just be strong Tim. It's only for a few months. So personally I never had any treats at all in that year.

There are a couple more meals I added to my list.

Paprika Pork

Ingredients

- low calorie cooking spray
- 2 large Spanish onions, cut into thin wedges
- 1 red pepper, deseeded and cut into chunks
- 500g lean pork fillet, cut into chunks
- 2 tbsp. paprika
- 300ml chicken or vegetable stock
- 6 tbsp. fat free natural yoghurt (unflavored yogurt)
- salt and freshly ground black pepper
- handful of roughly chopped fresh flat-leaf parsley (optional)

Method

1. Spray a large frying pan with low calorie cooking spray. Add the onions and pepper and cook for five to six minutes, stirring occasionally. Stir in the pork and cook for four minutes or until browned. Sprinkle over the paprika and cook for one minute. Add the stock to the pan and bring to the boil, then cover with a tightfitting lid and simmer for thirty minutes.

2. Stir most of the natural yogurt (unflavored yogurt) into the pork mixture and heat gently for two minutes. Season to taste, garnish with the remaining natural yogurt (unflavored yogurt) and parsley, if using, and serve with boiled rice and vegetables of your choice.

Tip: Pork tenderloin is very lean and the vacuum-packed kind offers the best value.

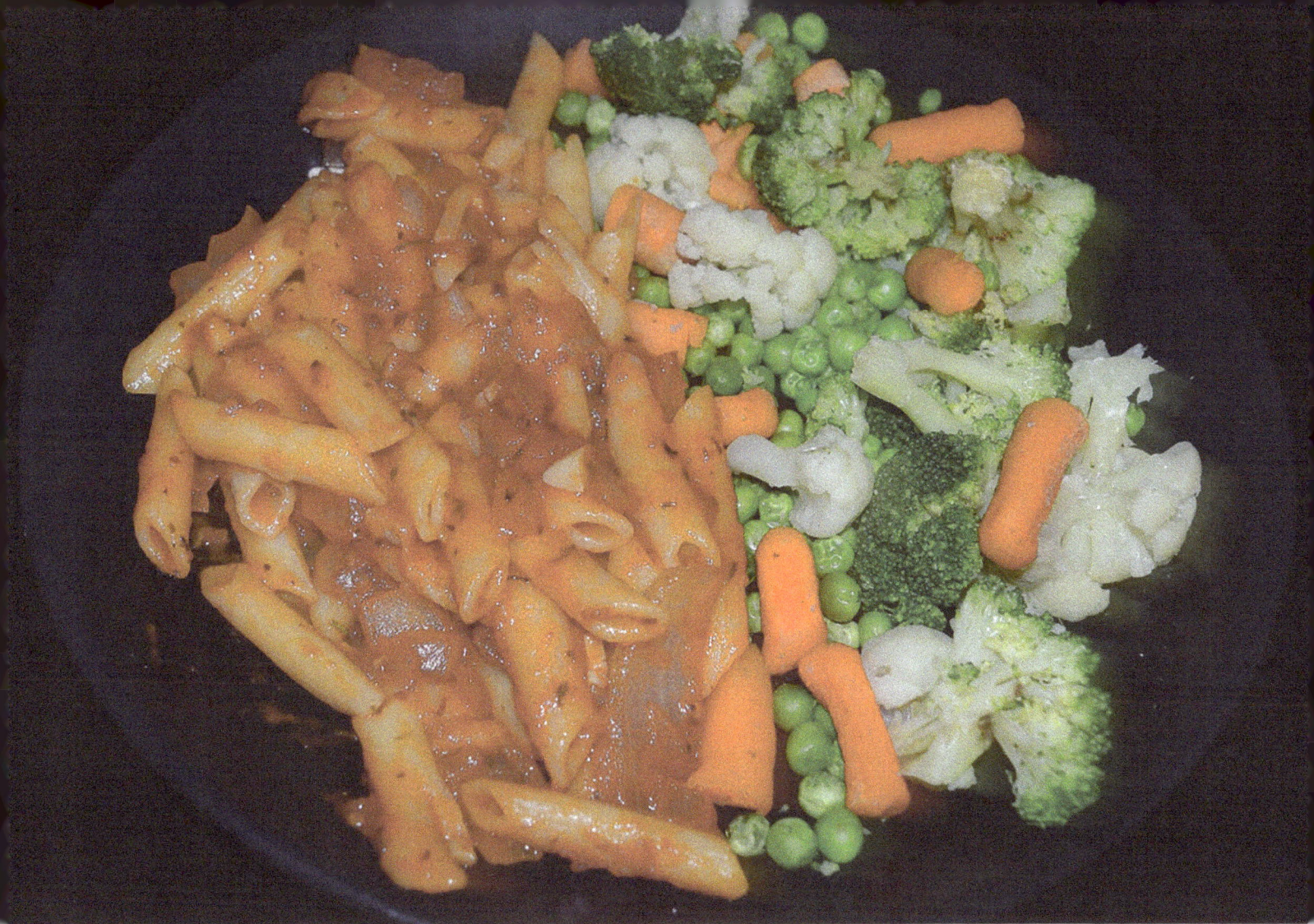

Pasta Arrabiata

Ingredients

- low calorie cooking spray
- 1 small onion, peeled and thinly sliced
- 3 garlic cloves peeled and crushed
- a pinch of dried mixed herbs
- 1 tsp. dried chili flakes
- 500g passata (tomato sauce)
- salt and freshly ground black pepper
- 500g penne pasta
- freshly chopped flat-leaf parsley, to garnish

Method

1. Spray a large saucepan with low calorie cooking spray and place over a medium heat. Cook the onion, garlic, herbs and chili flakes for four to five minutes. Stir in the passata and season to taste. Bring to the boil, cover and simmer for fifteen minutes, stirring occasionally.
2. Meanwhile, cook the pasta according to the packet instructions and drain. Add the pasta to the sauce and mix well. Garnish with chopped parsley and serve with a crisp green salad.

Tip: This sauce is also delicious using one or two finely chopped red chili peppers instead of the dried chili flakes. Make the sauce in advance and freeze until needed.

I used a lot more pasta in this meal and made the meal as a complete meal. You could use less pasta and have it with a crisp salad, vegetables, vegetables and couscous, a tin of beans and homemade chips (French fries), or like I have in the 2nd photo with sweet potato chips and 25g of grated cheese.

You can also try adding balsamic vinegar or Worcester sauce to give the sauce a little more of a kick. The amount of chili's you use is all down to you.

It's like all the meals in this book. There are many ways you can have these meals. It's all down to personal taste.

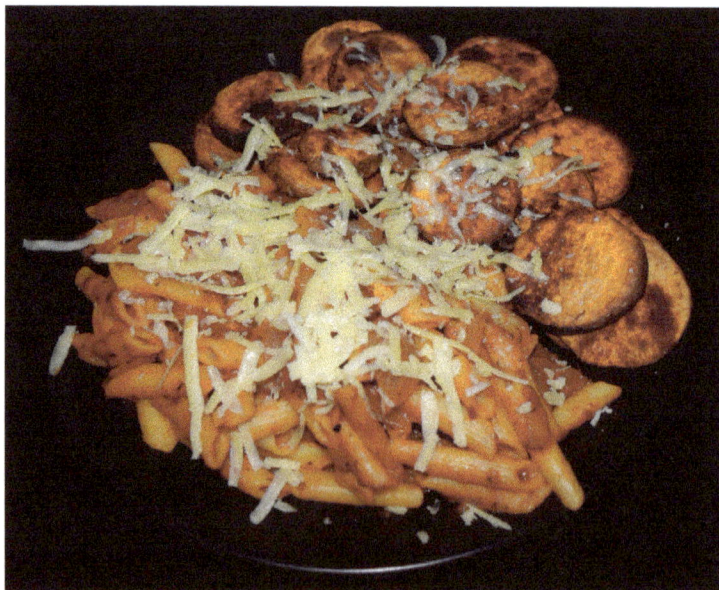

Savory Mince

Ingredients

- 250g 5% fat minced meat (ground beef)
- 2 large onions
- 4 large mushrooms
- 2 peppers
- 3 garlic cloves
- fresh ginger
- 300ml beef stock
- lots of worcester sauce (bold steak sauce)
- low calorie cooking spray

Method

Cut the mushrooms and peppers up and microwave them for five minutes. Chop the garlic, and cut the ginger up. Slice one onion very finely into small pieces and cut the other onion into quarters. Then fry all this in low calorie cooking spray. At the same time heat up the mince (ground beef). Mix 300ml of beef stock and add lots of Worcester sauce. When the onion has turned slightly brown, add it to the cooked mince and add the mushrooms and peppers. Pour on the beef stock and continue to cook for ten minutes. Then serve.

You can have savory mince with vegetables and couscous, salad or beans and homemade chips (French fries). It's a very versatile meal.

Beef Goulash

This Hungarian paprika-infused beef casserole is gorgeous when slow-cooked to release the fabulous meaty flavors.

Ingredients

- low calorie cooking spray
- 700g braising steak, all visible fat removed, cut into chunks
- 1 large onion, roughly chopped
- 400g mushrooms, sliced
- 2 garlic cloves, crushed
- 1½ tsp. paprika, plus a pinch to garnish
- 283g jar flame-roasted peppers in vinegar, drained and chopped
- 1 level tbsp. tomato purée
- 2 tbsp. beef concentrate
- 400g dried tagliatelle (pasta)
- ½ green cabbage, shredded
- 4 tbsp. fat-free yoghurt
- a small handful of fresh chives, chopped

Method

1. Preheat your oven to Gas Mark 5 – 375f.
2. Heat a frying pan sprayed with low calorie cooking spray and fry the beef until browned. Transfer to a flameproof casserole dish.
3. Spray the frying pan with more low calorie cooking spray and cook the onion for five minutes. Add the mushrooms and garlic and fry for five minutes, adding the paprika for the final minute. Add this to the casserole dish along with the peppers, tomato purée, beef concentrate and 275ml boiling water and stir over the heat until simmering. Cover and cook in the oven for two hours.

4. Cook the tagliatelle (pasta) according to package instructions and steam the cabbage for five minutes. Serve the goulash with the tagliatelle (pasta) and cabbage, topped with natural yogurt and sprinkled with chives and a pinch of paprika.

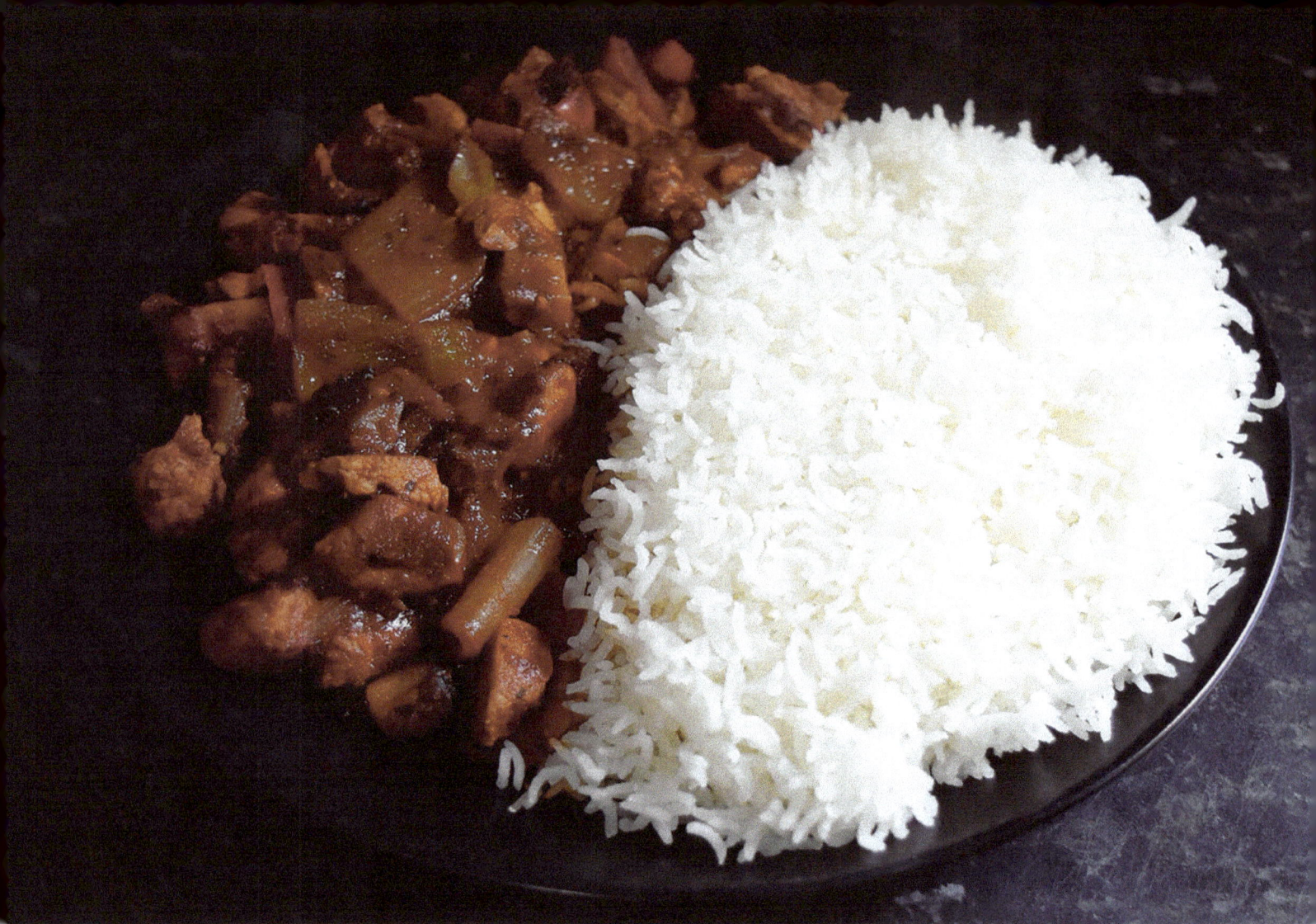

Diet Cola Chicken

This is actually called Diet Cola Chicken, but I don't use diet cola, I use chicken stock instead. It's Up to you which you use, diet cola or chicken stock. With either one it tastes fantastic.

Ingredients

- low calorie cooking spray
- 2 onions, 1 finely chopped and 1 cut into quarters
- 1 red pepper, 1 yellow and 1 green pepper, chopped into chunks
- 1 330ml Can Diet Cola
- 4 large mushrooms chopped into small pieces
- 4 garlic cloves, finely chopped
- 4 skinless chicken breasts, cut into pieces

- 2 tsp. worcester sauce (bold steak sauce)
- 4 tbsp. tomato purée
- 500g passata (tomato sauce) with onions and garlic
- 1 tbsp. dark soy sauce (kikkoman)
- 1 tsp. dried mixed herbs
- 330ml chicken stock

Method

1. Place a large pan sprayed with low calorie cooking spray over a high heat.
2. Microwave the peppers and mushrooms for five mins.
3. Fry the chicken.
4. Fry the onions, garlic and ginger until the onion is lightly browned. Add stock, passata (tomato sauce), tomato purée, garlic, Worcester sauce, soy sauce and dried mixed herbs to the chicken and stir well, then add the onions, peppers and mushrooms.
5. Bring to the boil, cover, reduce the heat to medium-low and simmer for twenty minutes. This reduces the sauce.

This is a very tasty meal you can have it with vegetables, salad, rice, pasta, mixed with couscous or even a tin of baked beans and homemade chips (French fries).

You can spice this meal up if you like and add chilli's. The Amount of balsamic vinegar and or Worcester sauce is completely down to your own individual taste.

This is a very versatile meal and very tasty.

My favourite meal.

At the end of the day all we want from our meals is 3 things. 1. Its filling. 2. It's tasty. 3. It's healthy. All the recipes in this book cover those 3 things. What more can anyone ask for from a meal. I've put in 29 recipes in this book. The truth is I could of put 200 recipes in this book. These recipes are to give you an idea on all the things you can cook. And because you are preparing these meals by yourself, you know what's going into the meals.

Eat, enjoy and lose weight

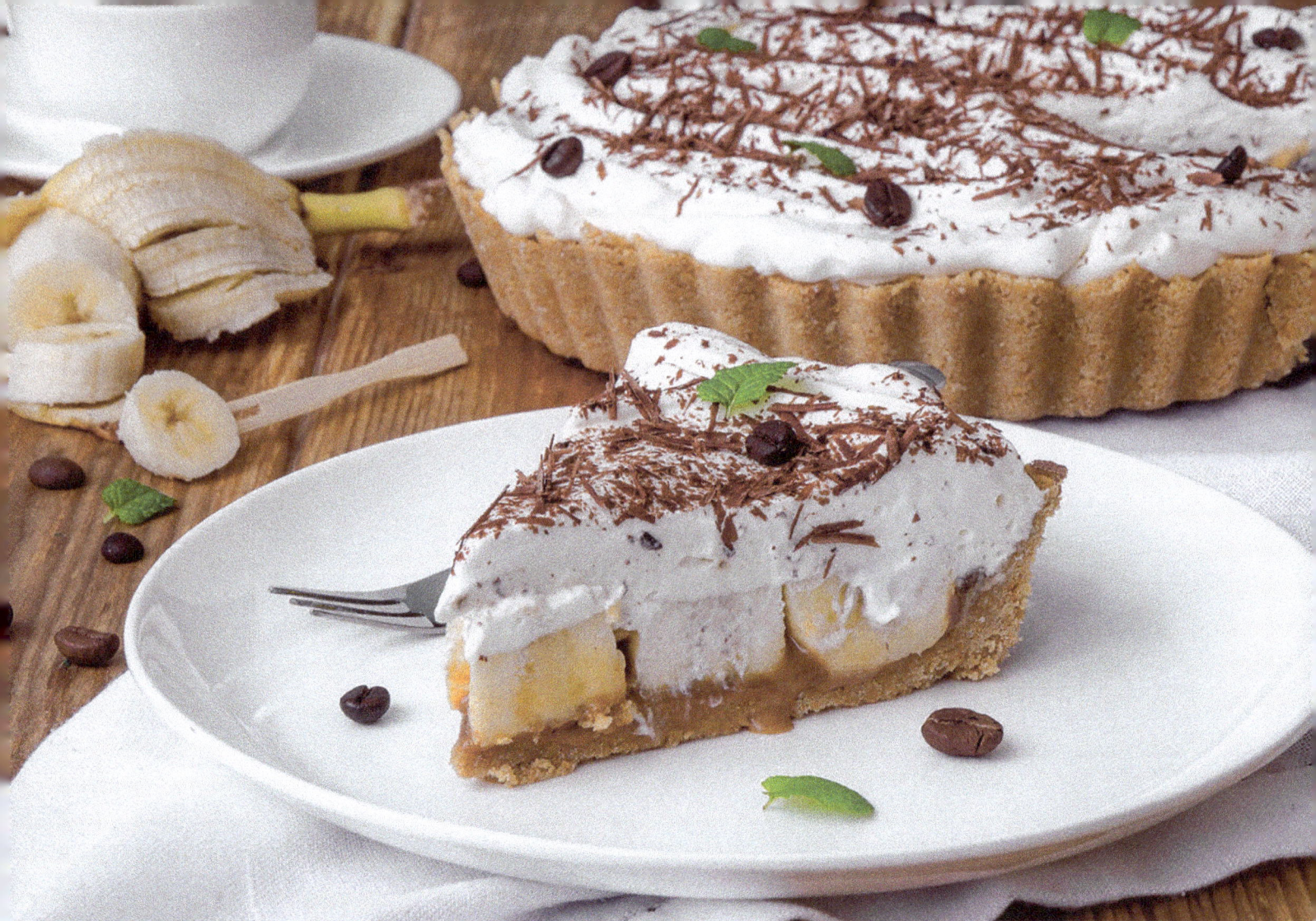

Banoffee Pie

Ingredients

- 10 reduced-fat digestive biscuits
- 5 level tbsp low-fat spread
- 2 x 12g sachets powdered gelatine
- 250g plain quark
- 3 x 175g pots Mullerlight Toffee yogurt (or any Free toffee yogurt)
- 3 level tbsp sweetener
- 1 tsp vanilla extract
- 2 egg whites*
- 2 bananas, thinly sliced
- Melted dark chocolate, to decorate (1½ Syns per level tsp), optional

Method

Preheat your oven to 190°C/fan 170°C/gas 5 and line a 20cm springform tin with baking parchment.

Place the biscuits in a polythene bag, finely crush with a rolling pin and tip into a bowl.

Melt the spread and add to the biscuits. Stir to mix well, then spoon into the prepared tin and press evenly over the base.

Bake in the oven for 15 minutes, then set aside to cool.

Dissolve the gelatine in 5 tbsp boiling water.

Whisk the quark in a bowl until smooth, then stir in the yogurt, sweetener and vanilla essence.

Whisk the egg whites until stiff and fold into the quark mixture with the gelatine liquid.

Spoon over the prepared biscuit base, smoothing the top with a palette knife, and chill for around 5 hours or until set.

Remove the pie from the tin and place on a serving plate. Arrange the banana slices neatly on top of the pie.

If you would like to decorate the pie with melted chocolate, drizzle it evenly over the top, remembering to count 1½ Syns per level teaspoon.

Cut the pie into 10 equal slices to serve.

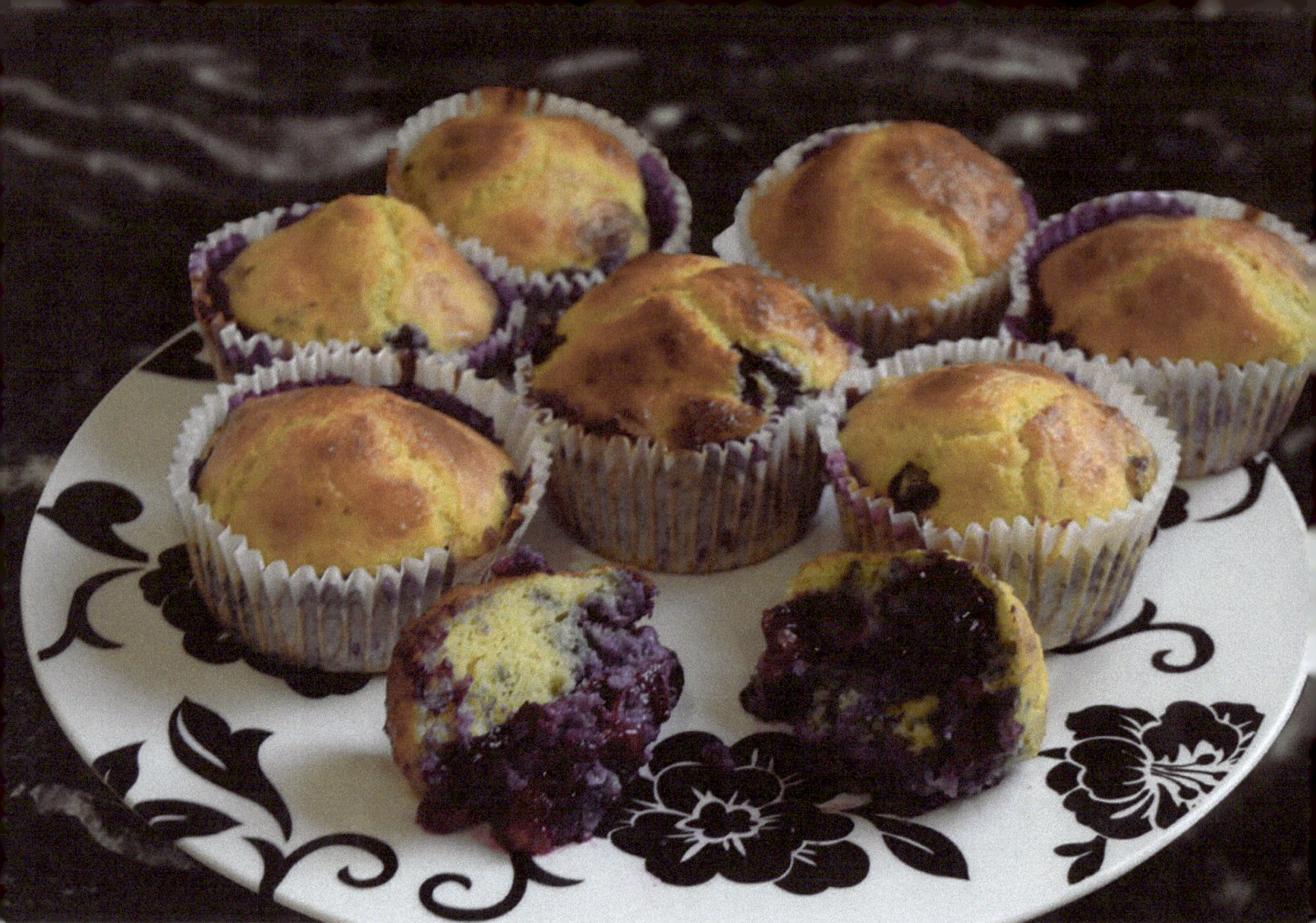

Blu Berry Muffins

- **Ingredients**
- 100g of plain all purpose flour
- 1 tsp of baking powder
- 1 pot of muller light
- 2 large eggs
- 1 tsp of vanilla extract
- 6 tbs of sweetener
- 80g of fresh blueberries
- cooking oil spray

Method

Preheat oven to 180c/350f (gas mark 4)

Add flour, eggs, yoghurt, sweetner, vanilla extract, cinnamon, baking powder, baking soda and whisk till all combined.

Add blueberries

Spray the muffin cases with low fat cooking spray and spoon the batter into the cases equally.

Place in the oven and bake for about 30-35 mins, they should be lightly golden.

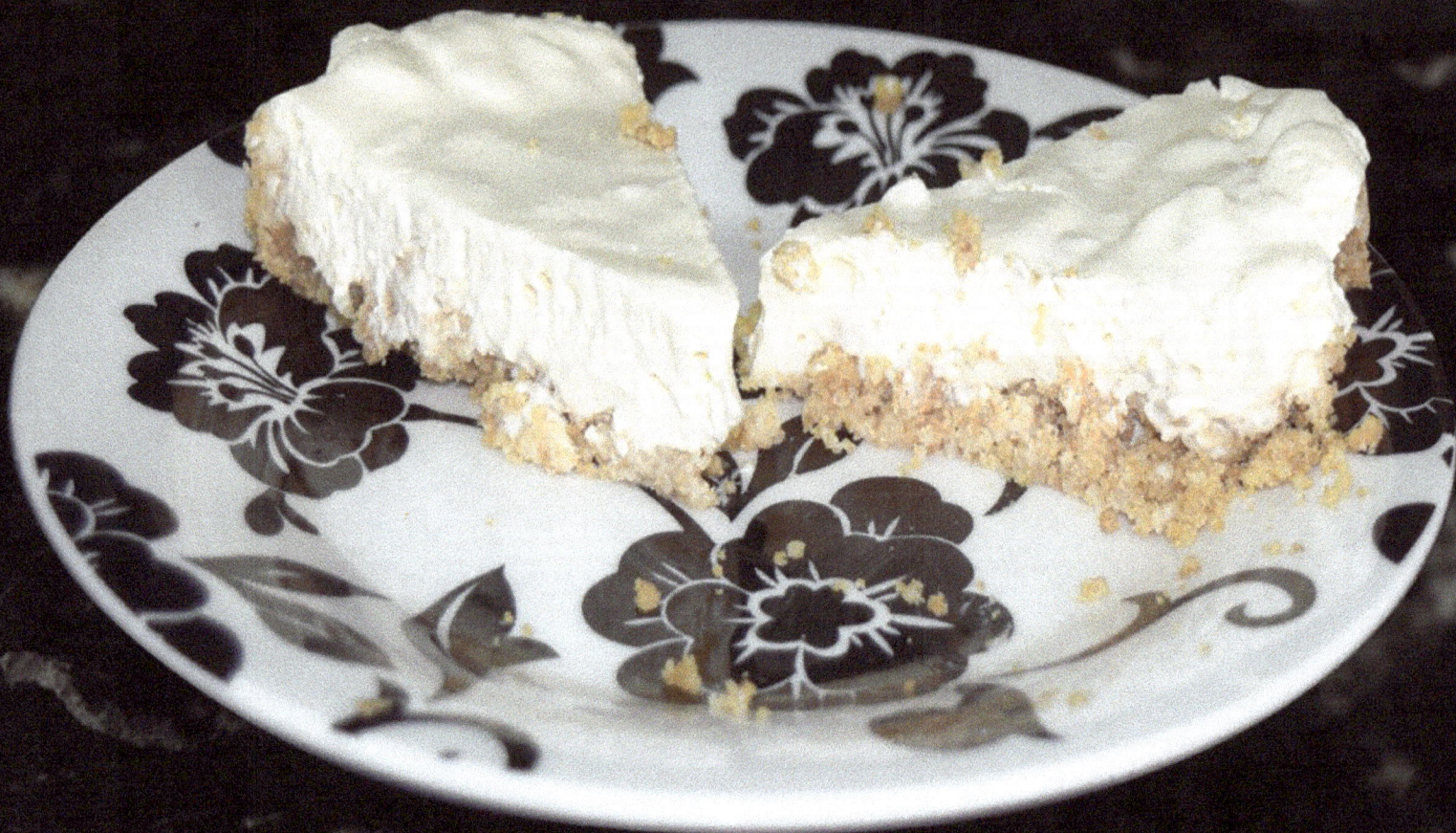

New York Style Cheesecake

Ingredients

- 80 g digestive biscuits *(28 syns)
- 40 g flora light margarine *(6 syns)
- 3 eggs
- 750 g vanilla quark *(=15 Syns in total)

Method

Preheat your oven on 200 degrees.

Butter the base of a 9 inch cake tin or similar and line with baking paper.

Blend the biscuits to crumbs and place in a mixing bowl.

Melt the margarine in a saucepan and stir in to the biscuit crumbs until mixed well.

Transfer the crumbs to the lined cake tin and press down with the back of a spoon.

In another mixing bowl, mix together the eggs and quark (and vanilla and sweetener if using plain quark).

Pour on top of the biscuit crumbs and smooth if needed to make level.

Place in the oven for 30-40 minutes until set, but if browning on the egdes too soon, cover the top with some tinfoil until the time is up.

Remove from the oven until cooled and place in the fridge until completely cold and serve.

Chapter Four

Stage Three

Okay, as I've said a few times, this book is about a lifestyle change; yes, that's true. However, I still considered this as a diet, for now. My mission was to lose all my excess weight.

Once my weight had gone I would still eat my food the same way by preparing and cooking all my own meals. But I'll be on a maintaining program.

I would like to point out that it's not essential that you go to the gym. What's essential is you prepare your own meals using natural ingredients.

It's May now and I've been on this food plan change now for five months. In that time I've lost 5 Stone (70 pounds).

For the last five months I've been having a breakfast each morning which is the first time in my life I've had a breakfast. For the last three months I've been having a lunch, which is also totally new to me. So I've been eating a lot more now than I have ever eaten, but I've lost 5 Stone (70 pounds). It reinforces the old adage, you are what you eat. It's not about how much you eat; it's about what you eat that matters.

I sincerely do hope that every reader is not just reading this book, but preparing the meals I've listed. By actually preparing these meals, you will begin to appreciate foods' values and the importance of what you are eating. By understanding the value in each food, you're making a conscious decision about what food you're eating. This is the lifestyle change.

By actually preparing your meals you're eating much healthier. When you lose any excess weight and you continue to eat the same, you will stay slim and healthy, adding years onto your lives. This surely has to be a good reason to change your lifestyle eating habits.

Okay, five months have gone and I want to change again. So I decided I'm going to cut out breakfast and lunch and just eat a lot more fruit during the day. I'm also going to go to the gym to increase my weight by adding muscle to my body. I want to change my body and put it into a better shape. This is done by hard work down at the gym.

To be honest I wasn't entirely sure this would work. I'd gotten into the habit of having a breakfast and a lunch, so I was unsure about taking those away. But I wanted to give it a try.

Now I'm going to the gym five times a week I'm going to have to increase my carbohydrates. Carbohydrates equal energy and I need energy because I'm going down to the gym now.

I had lost 5 Stone (70 pounds), so I wanted to add muscle to my body and put myself into a much better shape. I knew that by adding muscle this would slow my weight loss down, but it's something I wanted to do and try.

I bought a carbohydrate enriched protein drink. This was purely to increase my carbohydrates. I made sure I had potatoes or pasta with most of my evening meals, again to increase the carbohydrates.

I thought I'd try this out for a couple of weeks and check my weight to see what impact this major change had on me.

I had already lost 5 Stone (70 pounds). I wasn't entirely sure how much more weight I still had to lose, but it was clear I still needed to lose more weight. I felt this was the time as I was losing fat and I needed to add more muscle to my physique.

You Are What You Eat

I knew that because I had already lost 5 Stone (70 pounds) and I was now trying to build my muscles up it would slow my weight loss down by quite a bit. However I've come to the conclusion that it's not how much you weigh that matters it's how you feel inside.

If some of you are reading this and trying to lose weight as well, or if you ever come across a bad patch where you are struggling to focus or motivate yourself, do what I'd do. I would just ask myself, Tim, why are you on a diet? I'd use an image of myself with all my weight gone. Then I would tell myself I won't get to that image unless I work for it. This used to inspire me to continue.

Another great idea is to put your old jeans on. When you see how loose they are on you, you will be so happy and you can physically see the results of what you are doing.

I think we are all the same. When people come up to us and ask if we've lost weight, it makes us feel so much better. Keep up the good work all of you. You can and will achieve your weight loss.

Two weeks had gone by and I noticed my weight loss had slowed down. For the first few months I was losing on average about 5lbs per week. Now my weight loss was just under 2lbs per week. I put this down to the fact that I was trying to build my muscle size up and I was in fact gaining weight by going to the gym. But on the whole I was still losing my fat.

So I pushed on. I said to myself, okay Tim; give it a couple of months. I'd just keep checking my weight loss and body size.

Five Months Later of Going Down to the Gym

For five months I went down to the gym five times a week. I worked on a different body part each day, one body part per week. This is to maximize the buildup of a particular muscle. I was bodybuilding, trying to add muscle to myself, to give me a much better shape.

That's five months of eating tons of fruit during the day, and an evening meal. I'd have a carbohydrate enriched protein drink in the morning and afternoon just before training.

Most of my evening meals had potatoes or pasta in them because I needed to fuel my body with carbohydrates for the gym the next day.

Five months in and still losing weight is weird. Some weeks I'd lose no weight at all but still get smaller. My brain couldn't work it out. How could I not lose weight, yet get smaller?

It's been five months on Stage Three, five months of increased carbohydrates to help me build my muscle up. In those five months I still lost 3 Stone (42 pounds) and I've increased my muscle mass slightly. So it's been a success.

Chapter Five

Stage Four

This is probably my most crucial and dramatic stage of all. Ten months had passed now since I changed my lifestyle eating. I had lost 8 Stone in 10 months (112 pounds). I decided I needed an extra push now. My weight loss had slowed down because I had lost 8 Stone (112 pounds) and because I was going to the gym five times a week building my muscles up. When I first started my weight loss I was losing about 5 pounds a week. Now after ten months my weight loss was about 1 pound a week. So I decided I needed a big change.

So at the gym I would work extra hard on my cardiovascular exercise. Food wise I cut out carbohydrates completely. I was told by this bodybuilder who goes on shows that all professional body builders do the same thing. They strip the fat off their bodies before they go on shows. The way they do this is to do an intense cardiovascular workout and cut carbohydrates completely from their food intake.

The body screams out for carbohydrates after the intense workout. You give the body no carbohydrates at all so the body dives into the fat reserves to get the carbohydrates that it needs.

This is Stage Four of my planed weight loss. For Stage One I had a breakfast each morning, ate lots of fruit during the day and I had an evening meal. For Stage Two I had a breakfast each morning and a lunch. I still had fruit during the day but slightly less fruit. For Stage Three I cut out my breakfast and lunch, and had lots and lots of fruit during the day. I had two carbohydrate enriched protein drinks each day, I had potato or pasta with most of my evening meals and I went to the gym five times a week. In each stage I lost weight. Ten months had gone now and I've lost 8 Stone (112 pounds). It's been a remarkable success so far. Now time to start Stage Four.

As I said at the start of this chapter, Stage Four was definitely the most dramatic stage of all. I had already lost 8 Stone (112 pounds) and I had been going to the gym for five months to build up my muscle. However, during two months of Stage Four I lost an incredible 2 Stone (28 pounds). I was so shocked at how much I had lost in those two short months.

At Stage Four I was probably my most strict with my food intake. I ate tons and tons of fruit during the day and I had an evening meal. I cut out carbohydrates from my daily intake completely.

Yes, I was being extra strict with myself because I knew I was so close to the finish line. I told myself, hang in there Tim it will only be for a short time. I had already lost 8 Stone (112 pounds) and I was desperate to cross the finish line inside the year that I gave myself.

So in one year I'd lost 10 stone in weight (140 pounds). So in two short months I had lost 2 Stone (28 pounds) and that's after ten months of dieting and losing 8 Stone (112 pounds). I could still manage to lose 2 Stone (28 pounds) in two months. I was shocked at this result.

Okay, so now a year has gone by. I've lost 10 Stone (140 pounds), an amazing amount of weight to lose. If I had to be honest with you it was actually quite easy to do. I could see and feel the results of my food intake; this spurred me on to keep going. Having people come up to me and say how well I looked encouraged me to continue. The only real change I've done in the last year to what I have been doing for the last twenty years was to prepare my own meals. This one simple change in my eating had such a dramatic effect on me.

It affected my body size and I lost 10 stone (140 pounds) in weight. When I started one year ago, my waist was 52 inches. Now my waist is 33 inches; that's an incredible 19 inches lost off my waist in just one year. My shirt size a year ago was 5xl, now I'm wearing large shirts. I can actually walk into a normal shop and buy clothes to wear; I haven't been able to do this in over twenty years.

Just changing the way I eat my food has done this. These fantastic results are down to me preparing my own meals and making homemade sauces from natural ingredients.

None of you need to go on a complicated diet. None of you need to pay money to help you lose weight. None of you need to pay for any operations. All you need to do is to change your lifestyle eating. Prepare your own meals.

Mayonnaise, salad cream (miracle whip) and tomato ketchup are okay in small doses, nothing wrong with salad cream (miracle whip) on your salad. I've had that every week for a year and I lost 10 stone (140 pounds)

Obviously I don't need to tell you about sweets, crisps (potato chips), cakes and stuff like that.

This book is about a lifestyle change. The only thing you need to do is learn to prepare your own meals. Use natural ingredients in your meals and you will be fine. Prepackaged stuff is loaded with calories, chemicals and preservatives that you don't want or need.

Diet Over

I've not been on a diet for six months now. I still eat healthy; I still prepare my own meals. I'll continue to prepare my own meals forever now. It's so much healthier. I have changed my lifestyle eating.

Yes I do have the odd treat now and again, but I monitor my treats now. I have a chocolate bar, a cream cake, or a kebab, but that's okay; it's a treat. However I monitor my treats and I keep an eye on my weight.

A very big warning to all those who are overweight: you can never eat food like a normal person. Since you have stretched all your fat cells and molecules to an excess, with any slight food intake you will pile on the weight very quickly.

Now you have changed your lifestyle eating by preparing your own meals. This is for life.

Preparing your own meals is healthier for you.

You can lose weight.

You will look and feel better.

It will save you money.

It's Not How Much You Eat; It's What You Eat That Matters

You can make any meal tastier by adding herbs or spices; also you can add soy sauce or Worcester sauce and/or a homemade sauce.

You can make up your own sauces from natural ingredients. There are hundreds of homemade sauces if you Google them. Just check the ingredients and decide if you want to make that sauce.

You need to replace normal sugar with a sweetener sugar, like Canderel (Splenda) for example. There are many out there, either in tablet or normal sugar type to choose from.

My advice is to cut out bread completely is not needed, but go with wholemeal (wholegrain) if you need to.

Yes you can have treats like chocolate bars, crisps (potato chips), cakes, and ice-cream. All you need to do is to monitor your treats.

You can eat anything in moderation. Just be careful, that's all.

Since December 12th I now drink about three litres of water during the day. At night I drink black coffee or herbal tea and low calorie fizzy drinks, making it about five litres of water that I drink every day. This is very healthy for you to get into, drinking more water.

For the last seven months of my diet, I went to the gym five times a week. The first five months were just to try and build my muscles up and put some shape back into my body. For the last two months I still did the muscle workouts but I also did high intensity cardiovascular workouts while eating no carbohydrates at all. This was aimed at attacking the last remaining fat cells. It worked wonders; I lost 2 stone (28 pounds) in the last two months. I lost 10 stone (140 pounds) in a year.

I know not everyone can go to the gym, but to all those who can go to the gym, you can use the gym and this new way of eating to get fantastic results.

It doesn't matter if you go to the gym or not. Just by preparing your own meals using natural ingredients you can lose weight. Going to the gym will get you fitter, stronger and bigger. Going to the gym does not help you lose weight.

Everyone can lose weight if they prepare their own meals with fresh ingredients. Do not use a premade meals, or any prepackaged foods. No processed food and no ready to eat meals. Use only fresh ingredients. This way you are guaranteed to lose weight naturally.

Always remember it's not how much you eat, but what you eat that matters. Last year all my meals were very, very big, but I lost 10 stone (140 pounds) in one year.

Good luck to everyone trying to lose weight. It's not that hard, really. You just need to change your style of eating by preparing your own meals.

Chapter Six

Maintaining

Okay, last year I was on a diet. Okay, it wasn't really a diet; I was just eating healthily. But in my mind I told myself I was on a diet. In that year I lost 10 stone (140 pounds).

I have not been on a diet for six months now. I'm still eating my own cooked meals, but I have treats now and then. I just monitor my treats and keep an eye on my weight. In six months I haven't gained any weight. Okay, a couple of times I've eaten too many treats and put on some weight. Once I put on 1 stone (14 pounds) in weight. I didn't panic; I said okay, now I must just eat my own cooked meals for a couple of weeks with no treats at all to lose that little bit of weight. It worked.

I'm in a very good position now. I can have my treats and if I put a little weight on I am just strict on myself for a couple of weeks.

I'll never ever get fat again. I will still cook my own meals for the rest of my life. If everyone did this they can lose any excess weight.

I have not been on a diet for six months now and I still have not had any bread. I think I'm going to completely cut bread and butter out of my life altogether. There are too many calories for a single slice of bread. In my eyes it's not worth it. After one year and six months I've gotten used to my daily life without bread.

It's nothing complicated, nothing expensive, just common sense. Just cook your own meals with natural ingredients. Add any homemade sauce to add some flavor to your meals.

This is not a diet book. It's a lifestyle change book. It's not how much you eat but what you eat that matters. I cannot say this enough times. Every person on Earth can lose weight if they just prepare their own meals using natural ingredients. It's as simple as that.

I would like to point out that it's not essential that you go to the gym. What's essential is that you prepare your own meals using natural ingredients.

Good luck to everyone.

www.ingramcontent.com/pod-product-compliance
Lightning Source LLC
Chambersburg PA
CBHW042340030426
42335CB00030B/3416